घेरण्ड संहिता

Gheranda Samhita

(English Translation Accompanied by Sanskrit
Text in Roman Transliteration)

Translated into English by
Swami Vishnuswaroop

Published by

Divine Yoga Institute

Kathmandu, Nepal

Dedication

This book is dedicated to my Guru Swami Satyananda Saraswani,

Founder of Bihar School of Yoga,

Munger, India.

Swami Vishnuswaroop

Contents

Swami Vishnuswaroop

Gratitude

First of all I would like to express my heartfelt salutations to Adinatha (the Primordial Master) and my Guru Swami Satyananda Saraswati for their unwavering inspiration and guidance I have received for my work. I realize that my firm faith and belief in God and Guru is a motivational gift for me in completing this work. I could never have done it without their blessings.

I am always thankful to Ms. Bhawani Uprety for her untiring support she has provided me during my involvement in writing and translating various classical texts on yoga. My due thanks goes to her forever.

On the occasion of the Guru Purnima Day I wish that may God and Guru inspire us to tread the path of yoga in order to achieve the ultimate goal of human life!

- Swami Vishnuswaroop

Introduction

It is said that Gheraṇḍa Samhitā was composed in the Seventeenth Century by Sage Gheraṇḍa. Not so much is known regarding his time and place of birth. His system of yoga is called 'Saptāṅga Yoga' i.e. the yoga of seven limbs or parts. We know 'Aṣṭāṅga Yoga' (i.e. the eight limbs of yoga) by Sage Patañjali and 'Ṣaḍāṅga Yoga' (i.e. the six limbs of yoga) by Guru Gorakhanāth. All these systems of yoga with their specific limbs/parts are equally respected and followed in the yogic tradition.

The first aspect of yogic practice described in Gheraṇḍa Samhitā is ṣaṭkarma, the six yogic cleansing practices. Their practice is important to get rid of diseases from the body and purify it properly. The second aspect of yogic practice discussed is the āsana. The importance of āsana practice is that they help create firmness and stability in the body. The third aspect of practice described is the mudrā which is used to control the flow of prāṇa and retain and circulate it within the body. The fourth aspect of practice he talked is pratyāhāra.

According to Sage Gheraṇḍa, when body is purified through ṣaṭkarma, it is made firm and stable by āsana and prāṇa is controlled and retained by mudrā, then one can naturally do the practice of pratyāhāra. The fifth aspect of practice he taught is prāṇāyāma. In most of the prāṇāyāma practices he included mantras with them. Practice of pranayama with specific mantras creates direct impact on energy field within the body and mind through the vibrations of the mantras which eventually contribute for the expansion of awareness.

The sixth aspect of discourse in Gheraṇḍa Samhitā is dhyāna. The state of dhyāna arises naturally when the body is pure, firm and stable, prāṇa is controlled and the mind is withdrawn within itself. It describes three types of dhyāna for developing awareness and one-pointedness of the mind. The seventh and final aspect described in Gheraṇḍa Samhitā is samādhi. Its achievement is the final goal of yoga.

Publisher

Swami Vishnuswaroop

[2]

Chapter One

Discourse on Śaṭkarma

Salutations to Ādīśvara

आदीश्वराय प्रणमामि तस्मै येनोपदिष्टा हठयोगविद्या ।

विभ्राजते प्रोन्नतराजयोगमं आरोढुमिच्छोरधिरोहिणीव ॥

ādīśvarāya praṇamāmi tasmai

    yenopadiṣṭā haṭhayoga vidyā /

virājate pronnatarājayogaṃ

    āroḍhumicchādhirohiṇīva //

Salutation to *Śrī Ādinātha* (the primordial Lord *Śiva*) who imparted the knowledge of *Haṭha Yoga* that shines forth as a stairway for those who desire to climb highly advanced *Rāja Yoga*.

एकदा चण्डकापालिर्गत्वा घेरण्डकुट्टिरम् ।

प्रणम्य विनयाद्भक्त्या घेरण्डं परिपृच्छति ॥ १ ॥

ekadā caṇḍakāpālirgatvā gheraṇḍakuṭṭiram /

praṇamya vinayādbhaktayā gheraṇḍaṃ paripṛcchati //1//

One day *Caṇḍakapāli* went to the cottage of Sage *Gheraṇḍa*, saluted him with due respect and devotion and asked him. -1.

Body Based Yoga

चण्डकापालिरुवाच ।

घटस्थयोगं योगेश तत्त्वज्ञानस्य कारणम् ।

इदानीं श्रोतुमिच्छामि योगेश्वर वद प्रभो ॥२॥

caṇḍakapāliruvāca /

ghaṭasthayogaṃ yogeśa tattvajñānasya kāraṇam /

idānīṃ śrotumicchāmi yogeśvara vada prabho //2//

Caṇḍakapāli said: - O Lord of Yoga! I wish to learn *ghaṭasthayoga* (body based yoga) which is the cause of *tattvajñāna* (knowledge of the truth). O Lord of Yogīs! O Lord! Please tell me about it. -2.

घेरण्ड उवाच ।

साधु साधु महाबाहो यन्मां त्वं परिपृच्छसि ।

कथयामि च ते वत्स सावधानोऽवधारय ॥३॥

sādhu sādhu mahābāho yanmāṃ tvaṃ paripṛcchasi /

kathayāmi ca te vatsa sāvadhāno'vadhāraya //3//

Gheraṇḍa said: - O Mighty One! Well, you asked me. O child, I shall tell you. Listen to it very carefully. -3.

नास्ति मायासमः पाशो नास्ति योगात्परं बलम् ।

नास्ति ज्ञानात्परो बन्धुर्नाहङ्कारात्परो रिपुः ॥४॥

nāsti māyāsamaḥ pāśo nāsti yogātparaṃ balam /

nāsti jñānātparo bandhurnāhaṅkārārātparo ripuḥ //4//

There is no noose equal to *māyā* (illusion). There is no power equal to Yoga. There is no greater friend than *jñānā* (knowledge/wisdom). There is no greater enemy than *ahaṅkāra* (ego). -4.

अभ्यासात्कादिवर्णानां यथा शास्त्राणि बोधयेत् ।

तथा योगं समासाद्य तत्त्वज्ञानं च लभ्यते ॥५॥

abhyāsātkādivarṇānāṃ yathā śāstrāṇi bodhayet /

tathā yogaṃ samāsādya tattvajñānaṃ ca labhyate //5//

Just like by learning alphabets through practice all the *śāstrās* (branches of learning) are known, so by practicing yoga properly *tattvajñāna* (knowledge of the truth) is gained. -5.

सुकृतैर्दुष्कृतैः कार्यैर्जायते प्राणिनां घटः ।

घटादुत्पद्यते कर्म घटीयन्त्रं यथा भ्रमेत् ॥६॥

sukṛtairduṣkṛtaiḥ kāryairjāyate prāṇināṃ ghaṭaḥ /

ghaṭādutpadyate karma ghaṭīyantraṃ yathā bhramet //6//

The physical bodies of all creatures are produced as the result of their good or bad actions. The karma (action) is originated from the body and its cycle continues just like the circle of a *ghaṭīyantra* (water-wheel). -6.

ऊर्ध्वार्धो भ्रमते यद्वद्घटीयन्त्रं गवां वशात् ।

तद्वत्कर्मवशाज्जीवो भ्रमते जन्ममृत्युभिः ॥७॥

urdhvārdho bhramate yadvatghaṭīyantraṃ gavāṃ vaśāt/

tadvatkarmavaśājjīvo bhramate janmamṛtyubhiḥ //7//

Just like the water-wheel goes up and down as it is moved by the bullocks, so the *jīva* (the embodied Self) goes through the cycle of birth and death due to its (past) karma. -7.

आमं कुम्भमिवाम्भस्थो जीर्यमाणः सदा घटः ।

योगानलेन सन्दह्य घटशुद्धिं समाचरेत् ॥८॥

āmakumbha ivāmbhastho jīryamāṇaḥ sadā ghaṭaḥ /

yogānalena sandahyā ghaṭaśuddhiṃ samācaret //8//

Like a raw clay pot filled with water is destroyed (as it melts quickly), so the body is always deteriorated soon. One should purify the body baking it well by the fire of yoga. -8.

The Seven Means of Purification

शोधनं दृढता चैव स्थैर्यं धैर्यं च लाघवम् ।

प्रत्यक्षं च निर्लिप्तं च घटस्थसप्तसाधनम् ॥९॥

śodhanaṃ dṛḍhatā caiva

      sthairyaṃ dhairyaṃ ca lāghavam /

pratyakṣaṃ ca nirliptaṃ ca

      ghaṭasthasaptasādhanam //9//

The seven means of cleaning the physical body are: - purification, firmness, stability, endurance, lightness, direct knowledge and total detachment (from the world). -9.

षट्कर्मणा शोधनं च आसनेन भवेद्दृढम् ।

मुद्रया स्थिरता चैव प्रत्याहारेण धीरता ॥१०॥

प्राणायामाल्लाघवं च ध्यानात्प्रत्यक्षमात्मनः ।

समाधिना निर्लिप्तं च मुक्तिरेव न संशयः ॥११॥

ṣaṭkarmaṇā śodhanaṃ ca āsanena bhaveddṛḍham /

mudrayā sthiratā caiva pratyāhāreṇa dhīratā //10//

prāṇāyāmāllāghavaṃ ca dhyānātpratyakṣamātmanaḥ /

samādhinā nirliptaṃ ca muktireva na saṃśayaḥ //11//

The purification is achieved through the practice of *ṣaṭkarma* (the six yogic cleansing practices); firmness through *āsanas*; stability through *mudrās*; endurance through *pratyāhāra*; lightness (of the body) through *prāṇāyāma*; direct knowledge through *dhyāna*; and total detachment (from the world) through *samādhi* which is certainly *mukti* (liberation) without any doubt. -10-11.

The Six Cleansing Practices

धौतिर्बस्तिस्तथा नेतिनौंलिकी त्राटकं तथा ।

कपालभातिश्चैतानि षट्कर्माणि समाचरेत् ॥१२॥

dhautirvastistathā netiḥ laulikī trāṭakaṃ tathā /

kapālabhātiścetāni ṣaṭkarmāṇi samācaret //12//

The *ṣaṭkarmas* to be practiced are *dhauti, vasti, neti, laulika, trāṭaka* and *kapālabhāti*. -12.

अन्तर्धौतिर्दन्तधौतिर्हृद्धौतिर्मूलशोधनम् ।

धौतिं चतुर्विधां कृत्वा घटं कुर्वन्ति निर्मलम् ॥१३॥

antardhautirdantadhautirhṛddhutirmūlaśodhanam /

dhautiṃ caturvidāṃ kṛtvā ghaṭaṃ kurvanti nirmalam //13//

Antardhauti (internal cleansing), *dantadhauti* (cleaning of teeth), *hṛddhuti* (cleaning of the heart i.e. the gullet, the lungs and the stomach) and *mūlaśodhana* (cleaning of the rectum) are the four kinds *dhautis* which purify the physical body. -13.

The Internal Cleansing

वातसारं वारिसारं वह्निसारं बहिष्कृतम् ।

घटस्य निर्मलार्थाय ह्यन्तधौंतिश्चतुर्विधा ॥१४॥

vātasāraṃ vārisāraṃ vanhisāraṃ bahiṣkṛtam //

ghaṭasya nirmalārthāya antardhutiścaturvidhā //14//

There are four types of *antardhauti* for the purification of the physical body. They are: - *vātasāra* (purification by air), *vārisāra* (purification by water), *vanhisāra* (purification by fire) and *bahiṣkṛta* (expulsion through rectum). -14.

Vātasāra Dhauti

काकचञ्चूवदास्येन पिबेद्वायुं शनैः शनैः ।

चालयेदुदरं पश्चाद्वर्त्मना रेचयेच्छनैः ॥१५॥

kākacañcuvadāsyena pibedvāyuṃ śanaiḥ śanaiḥ /

cālayedudaraṃ pascadvartmanā recayecchanaiḥ //15//

Inhale the air slowly through the mouth like a beak of a crow, fill the stomach and move the abdomen, and then slowly expel the air moving out through the downward passage. -15.

वातसारं परं गोप्यं देहनिर्मलकारणम् ।

सर्वरोगक्षयकरं देहानलविवर्धकम् ॥१६॥

vātasāraṃ paraṃ gopyaṃ deha nirmalakārakam /

sarva rogakṣayakaraṃ dehānalavivardhakam //16//

Vātasāra is a highly secret practice. It is the purifier of the physical body. It destroys all diseases and increases digestive fire. -16.

Vārisāra Dhauti

आकण्ठं पूरयेद्वारि वक्त्रेण च पिबेच्छनैः ।

चालयेदुदरेणैव चोदराद्रेचयेदधः ॥१७॥

ākaṇṭhaṃ pūrayedvāri vaktreṇa ca pibetcchanaiḥ /

cālayeddudareṇaiva codarādrecayedadhaḥ //17//

Drink the water through the mouth filling up to the throat, drink it slowly; and move it through the abdomen and then expel it forcibly through the rectum. -17.

वारिसारं परं गोप्यं देहनिर्मलकारकम् ।

साधयेद्यः प्रयत्नेन देवदेहं प्रपद्यते ॥ १८ ॥

vārisāraṃ paraṃ gopyaṃ dehanirmalakārakam /

sādhayettatprayatnena devadehaṃ prapadyate //18//

Vārisāra is a highly secret practice. It is the purifier the body. One who carefully practices it, his body is transformed into a divine body. -18.

वारिसारं परां धौतिं साधयेद्यः प्रयत्नतः ।

मलदेहं शोधयित्वा देवदेहं प्रपद्यते ॥ १९ ॥

vārisāraṃ parāṃ dhautiṃ sādhayedyaḥ prayatnataḥ /

maladehaṃ sodhayitvā devadehaṃ prapadyate //19//

Vārisāra is the best *dhauti*. One who practices it carefully purifies the impurities of his body and transforms it into the *devadeha* (divine body). -19.

Agnisāra

नाभिग्रन्थिं मेरुपृष्ठे शतवारं च कारयेत् ।

उदरामयजं त्यक्त्वा जाठराग्निं विवर्धयेत् ॥ २० ॥

nābhigranthiṃ merupṛṣṭhe śatavāraṃ ca kārayet /

agnisārameṣā dhautiryogināṃ yogasiddhidā //20//

Pull in the navel knot (center) towards the spinal column and then push out one hundred times. This is *agnisaradhauti* which gives perfection in yoga. -20.

अग्निसारमियं धौतिर्योगिनां योगसिद्धिदा ।

एषा धौतिः परा गोप्या देवानामपि दुर्लभा ।

केवलं धौतिमात्रेण देवदेहो भवेद्ध्रुवम् ॥२१॥

udarāmayajaṃ tyaktvā jaṭharāgniṃ vivardhayet /

eṣā dhautiḥ parā gopyā devānāmapi durlabhā /

kevalaṃ dhautimātreṇa devadeho bhaveddhruvam //21//

By its practice all diseases of the stomach are cured and digestive fire is increased. This *dhauti* should be kept highly secret, and it is difficult to attain even by gods. One certainly gets a divine body through the practice of this *dhauti* alone. -21.

Bahiṣkṛta Dhauti

काकीमुद्रां साधयित्वा पूरयेदुदरं मरुत् ।

धारयेदर्धयामं तु चालयेदधोवर्त्मना ।

एषा धौतिः परा गोप्या न प्रकाश्या कदाचन ॥२२॥

kākīmudrāṃ śādhayitvā pūrayedudaraṃ marut /

dhārayedardhayāmaṃ tu cālayedadhovartmanā /

eṣā dhautiḥ parā gopyā na prakāśyā kadācana //22//

Fill the stomach with air through the practice of *kākīmudrā*, hold it there for one and a half hours, and then force it to move downwards. This *dhauti* should be kept highly secret and not to be disclosed to anyone. -22.

Prakṣālana

[10]

नाभिदग्ने जले स्थित्वा शक्तिनाडीं विसर्जयेत् ।

कराभ्यां क्षालयेन्नाडीं यावन्मलविसर्जनम् ।

तावत्प्रक्षाल्य नाडीं च उदरे वेशयेत्पुनः ॥२३॥

nābhimagnajale sthitvā śaktināḍīṃ visarjayet /

karābhyāṃ kṣālayennāḍīṃ yāvanmalavisarjanam /

tāvatprakṣālya nāḍīṃ ca udare viśayetpunaḥ //23//

Stand in navel-deep water, gently draw out *śaktināḍī* (the intestine) and carefully wash it with the hands until it is clean and then draw it back again into the abdomen. -23.

इदं प्रक्षालनं गोप्यं देवानामपि दुर्लभम् ।

केवलं धौतिमात्रेण देवदेहो भवेद्ध्रुवम् ॥२४॥

idaṃ prakṣālanaṃ gopyaṃ devānāmapi durlabham /

kevalaṃ dhautimātreṇa devadeho bhavet dhruvam //24//

This *prakṣālana* (washing practice) should be kept secret. It is difficult to attain even by gods. Through this practice alone one certainly obtains a divine body. -24.

यामार्धधारणाशक्ति यावन्न साधयेन्नरः ।

बहिष्कृतं महद्धौतिस्तावच्चैव न जायते ॥२५॥

yamārdha dhāraṇāśaktiṃ yāvanna dhārayennarah /

bahiṣkṛtaṃ mahaddhautistāvaccaiva na jāyate //25//

As long as one does not have the power of retaining the breath for one and half hours, so long he should not attempt to do *bahiṣkṛta dhauti*, the great purification practice. -25.

Dantadhauti

दन्तमूलं जिह्वामूलं रन्ध्रं च कर्णयुग्मयोः ।

कपालरन्ध्रं पञ्चैते दन्तधौतिं विधीयते ॥२६॥

dantamūlaṃ jihvāmūlaṃ randhraṃ karṇayugmayoḥ /

kapālarandhraṃ pañcaite dantadhautirvidhīyate //26//

Purification of the root of the teeth, the root of the tongue, the two holes of the ears (counted as two cleaning practices) and the frontal sinuses are known as five kinds *dantadhauti*. -26.

खादिरेण रसेनाथ मृत्तिकया च शुद्धया ।

मार्जयेद्दन्तमूलं च यावत्किल्बिषमाहरेत् ॥२७॥

khādireṇa rasenātha śuddhamṛttikayā tathā /

mārjayeddantamūlaṃ ca yāvaṭkilviṣamāharet//27//

Rub the root of the teeth with catechu powder/juice or with pure earth until the impurities are removed. -27.

दन्तमूलं परा धौतिर्योगिनां योगसाधने ।

नित्यं कुर्यात्प्रभाते च दन्तरक्षाय योगवित् ।

दन्तमूलं धावनादिकार्येषु योगिनां मतम् ॥२८॥

dantamūlaṃ parādhutiryogināṃ yoga sādhane /

nityaṃ kuryātprabhāte ca dantarakṣāṃ ca yogavit /

dantamūlaṃ dhāvanādikāryeṣu yogināṃ matam //28//

The cleaning the root of teeth is a great *dhauti* for yogīs in their yogic *sādhanā* (practice). It should be done regularly in the morning for the protection of the teeth. The knowers of yoga regard that this *dhauti* is one of the important acts of yogīs like their other practices. -28.

Jihvā Dhauti

अथातः संप्रवक्ष्यामि जिह्वाशोधन कारणम् ।

जरामरणरोगादीन्नाशयेद्दीर्घलम्बिका ॥२९॥

athātaḥ sampravakṣyāmi jihvāśodhana kāraṇam /

jarāmaraṇarogādīnnāśayeddīrghalambikā //29//

Now I shall explain you about the reason of cleaning the tongue. This practice of *dīrghalambikā* (elongation of the tongue) destroys old age, death and disease, etc. -29.

तर्जनीमध्यमानामा अङ्गुलित्रययोगतः ।

वेशयेद्गलमध्ये तु मार्जयेल्लम्बिकामूलम् ।

शनैः शनैर्मार्जयित्वा कफदोषं निवारयेत् ॥३०॥

tarjanīmadhyamānāmā aṅgulitrayayogataḥ /

veśayedgalamadhye tu mārjayellambikāmūlam /

śanaiḥ śanaiḥ mārjayitvā kaphadoṣaṃ nivārayet //30//

Insert the index, middle and ring fingers jointly into the throat, rub and clean well the root of the tongue and remove the imbalance of *kapha* (phlegm) rubbing and cleaning it slowly and regularly. -30.

मार्जयेन्नवनीतेन दोहयेच्च पुनः पुनः ।

तदग्रं लोहयन्त्रेण कर्षयित्वा शनैः शनैः ॥३१॥

mārjayennavanītena dohayecca punaḥ punaḥ /

tadagraṃ lohayantreṇa karṣayitvā śanaiḥ śanaiḥ //31//

Having the tongue cleaned, rub it with butter and milk it again and again. Then holding the tip of the tongue with an iron tongs, pull it out slowly and slowly. -31.

नित्यं कुर्यात्प्रयत्नेन रवेरुदयकेऽस्तके ।

एवं कृते च नित्यं सा लम्बिका दीर्घतां व्रजेत् ॥३२॥

nityaṃ kuryātprayatnena raverudayake'stake /

evaṃ kṛte ca nityaṃ sā lambikā dīrghatāṃ vrajet //32//

It should be done carefully everyday at the time of rising and setting of the sun. In this way, through regular practice the tongue becomes longer. -32.

Karṇa Dhauti

तर्जन्यङ्गुल्य काग्रेण मार्जयेत्कर्णरन्ध्रयोः ।

नित्यमभ्यासयोगेन नादान्तरं प्रकाशयेत् ॥३३॥

tarjanyanāmikā yogānmārjayet karṇarandhrayoḥ /

nityamabhyāsa yogena nādāntaraṃ prakāśayet //33//

The holes of the ears should be cleaned with the index and/or ring fingers. The inner mystical sounds become evident through the regular practice of this yogic method. -33.

Kapālarndhra Dhauti

वृद्धाङ्गुष्ठेन दक्षेण मर्दयेद्भालरन्ध्रकम् ।

एवमभ्यासयोगेन कफदोषं निवारयेत् ॥३४॥

vṛddhāṅgusṭhena dakṣeṇa mārjayedbhālarandhrakam /

evamabhyāsayogena kaphadoṣaṃ nivārayet //34//

The top opening of the head should be patted with the thumb of the right hand. The imbalance of *kapha* is removed through the practice of this yogic method. -34.

नाडी निर्मलतां याति दिव्यदृष्टिः प्रजायते ।

निद्रान्ते भोजनान्ते च दिवान्ते च दिने दिने ॥३५॥

nāḍī nirmalatām yāti divyadṛṣṭiḥ prajāyate /

nidrānte bhojanānte ca divānte ca dine dine //35//

The *nāḍīs* (*prānic* channels) become pure (by this practice) and *divyadṛṣṭi* (clairvoyance) is achieved. It should be practiced daily at the end of sleep, at the end of meals, and at the end of the day. -35.

Hṛddhauti

हृद्धौतिं त्रिविधां कुर्याद्दण्डवमनवाससा ॥३६॥

hṛddhautiṃ trividhāṃ kuryāddaṇḍavamanavāsasā //36//

There are three kinds *hṛddhauti* (cleaning of the heart): - *daṇḍadhauti* (cleaning by using stalk), *vamanadhauti* (cleaning by vomiting) and *vāsadhauti* (cleaning by using cloth). -36.

रम्भादण्डं हरिद्दण्डं वेत्रदण्डं तथैव च ।

हन्मध्ये चालयित्वा तु पुनः प्रत्याहरेच्छनैः ॥३७॥

rambhādaṇḍaṃ hariddaṇḍaṃ vetradaṇḍaṃ tathaiva ca /

hṛnmadhye cālayitvā tu punaḥ pratyāharecchanaiḥ //37//

Use a stalk of the soft part of a banana plant or a stalk of the turmeric or a stalk of cane and insert it into the gullet and move it there (several times) and then take it out slowly. -37.

कफपित्तं तथा क्लेदं रेचयेदूर्ध्ववर्त्मना ।

दण्डधौतिविधानेन हृद्रोगं नाशयेद्ध्रुवम् ॥३८॥

kaphaṃpittaṃ tathā kledaṃ recayedūrdhvavartmanā /

daṇḍadhautividhānena hṛdrogaṃ nāśayet dhruvam //38//

The phlegm, bile and other watery impurities should be expelled out through the opening of the mouth. The heart disease is certainly destroyed by the proper practice of this *daṇḍadhauti*. -38.

Vamanadhauti

भोजनान्ते पिबेद्वारि चाकण्ठं पूरितं सुधीः ।

ऊर्ध्वीं दृष्टिं क्षणं कृत्वा तज्जलं वमयेत्पुनः ।

नित्यमभ्यासयोगेन कफपित्तं निवारयेत् ॥३९॥

bhojanānte pibetvāri cākaṇṭhaṃ pūritaṃ sudhiḥ /

urdhvā dṛṣṭiṃ kṣaṇaṃ kṛtvā tatjalaṃ vamayetpunaḥ /

nityamabhyāsayogena kaphapittaṃ nivārayet //39//

The wise practitioner at the end of his meal should drink water filling up to the throat and looking upwards for a short time should vomit up the water. The *kapha* (phlegm) and *pitta* (bile) are cured through this regular yogic practice. -39.

Vāsadhauti

चतुरङ्गुल विस्तारं सूक्ष्मवस्त्रं शनैर्ग्रसेत् ।

पुनः प्रत्याहरेदेतत्प्रोच्यते धौतिकर्मकम् ॥४०॥

caturaṅgula vistāraṃ sukṣmavastraṃ śanairgraset /

punaḥ pratyāharedetatprocyate dhautikarmakam //40//

Slowly swallow a thin cloth having the width of four fingers and slowly take it out. This is called *vāsa/vastradhauti*. -40.

गुल्मज्वरप्लीहाकुष्ठकफपित्तं विनश्यति ।

आरोग्यं बलपुष्टिश्च भवेत्तस्य दिने दिने ॥४१॥

gulmajvaramlaplīhakuṣṭhakaphapittaṃ vinasyati /

ārogyaṃ balapuṣṭiśca bhavettasya dine dine //41//

The practice of this *dhauti* cures enlarged glands and spleen, fever, leprosy and *kapha* and *pitta* related disorders. Good health, strength and nourishment are gradually acquired through this practice. -41.

Mūlaśodhana

अपानक्रूरता तावद्यावन्मूलं न शोधयेत् ।

तस्मात्सर्वप्रयत्नेन मूलशोधनमाचरेत् ॥४२॥

apānakrūratā tāvadyāvanmūlaṃ na śodhayet /

tasmātsarvaprayatnena mūlaśodhanamācaret //42//

The *apānakrūratā* (the cruelty of *apāna vāyu*) cannot be eliminated unless the rectum is not purified. Therefore, purification of the rectum should be done with all effort. -42.

पीतमूलस्य दण्डेन मध्यमाङ्गुलिनाऽपि वा ।

यत्नेन क्षालयेद्गुह्यं वारिणा च पुनः पुनः ॥४३॥

pītamūlasya daṇḍena madhyamāṅgulinā'pi vā /

yatnena kṣālayetguhyaṃ vāriṇā ca punaḥ punaḥ //43//

The rectum should be carefully cleaned by means of a turmeric stalk or the middle finger with water again and again. -43.

वारयेत्कोष्ठकाठिन्यमामाजीर्णं निवारयेत् ।

कारणं कान्तिपुष्ट्योश्च दीपनं वह्निमण्डलम् ॥४४॥

vārayetkoṣṭhakāṭhinyamāmājīrṇa nivārayet /

kāraṇaṃ kāntipuṣṭyocca dīpanaṃ vanhimaṇḍalam //44//

The practice of *mūlaśodhana*destroys constipation, indigestion and digestive disorders. It increases the beauty and vitality of the body and activates the digestive fire. -44.

Vasti

जलवस्तिः शुष्कवस्तिर्वस्ति च द्विविधौ स्मृतौ ।

जल वर्स्ति जले कुर्याच्छुष्कवर्स्ति सदा क्षितौ ॥४५॥

jalavastiḥ śuṣkavastirvasti ca dvividhau smṛtā /

jala vastiṃ jale kuryācchuṣkavastiṃ sadā kṣitau //45//

The *vasti* is considered of two kinds: - *jala vasti* and *śuṣka vasti*. *Jala vasti* is practiced in water and *śuṣka vasti* is always practiced on land. -45.

Jala vasti

नाभिमग्नजले पायुं न्यस्तवानुत्कटासनम् ।

आकुञ्चनं प्रसारं च जल बर्स्ति समाचरेत् ॥४६॥

nābhimagnajale pāyuṃ nyastavānutkaṭāsanam /

ākuñcanaṃ prasāraṃ ca jala vastiṃ samācaret //46//

Go into water up to the navel deep and perform *utkaṭāsana*. Then contract and expand the anus muscles for the practice of *jala vasti*. -46.

प्रमेहं च उदावर्तं क्रूरवायुं निवारयेत् ।

भवेत्स्वच्छन्ददेहश्च कामदेवसमो भवेत् ॥४७॥

pramehaṃ ca udāvartaṃ krūravāyuṃ nivārayet /

bhavetsvacchandadehaśca kāmadeva samo bhavet //47//

This practice cures *prameha* (diabetes), *udāvarta* (digestive disorders) and *krūravāyu* (severe disorders of the *vāyu*). The body becomes free from all restraints and one attains the beauty equal to *kāmadeva* (the god of love). -47.

Sthala Vasti

बर्सि पश्चिमोत्तानेन चालयित्वा शनैरधः ।

अश्विनीमुद्रया पायुमाकुञ्चयेत्प्रसारयेत् ॥४८॥

paścimottānato vastiṃ cālayitvā śanaiḥ śanaiḥ /

aśvinīmudrayā pāyumākuñcayetprasārayet //48//

After assuming the *paścimottānāsana*, move the intestines slowly in the lower region and then contract and expand the anus muscles through the practice of *aśvinīmudrā*. -48.

एवमभ्यासयोगेन कोष्ठदोषो न विद्यते ।

विवर्धयेज्जठराग्निमामवातं विनाशयेत् ॥४९॥

evamabhyāsayogena koṣṭhadoṣo na vidyate /

vivarddhayejjaṭharāgnimāmavātaṃ vināśayet //49//

Thus, constipation does not exist through this yogic practice. The digestive fire is increased and flatulence is destroyed. -49.

Neti

वितस्तिमानं सूक्ष्मसूत्रं नासानाले प्रवेशयेत् ।

मुखान्निर्गमयेत्पश्चात्प्रोच्यते नेतिकर्मकम् ॥५०॥

vitastimānaṃ sūkṣmasūtraṃ nāsānale praveśayet /

mukhānnirgamayetpaścāt procyate netikarmakam //50//

Insert into the nostril a thin thread about ten-inch long and then it should be taken out through the mouth. This is called *neti karma*. -50.

साधनान्नेतिकार्यस्य खेचरीसिद्धिमाप्नुयात् ।

कफदोषा विनश्यन्ति दिव्यदृष्टिः प्रजायते ॥५१॥

sādhanānnetikāryasya khecarisiddhimāpnuyāt /

kaphadoṣā vinasyanti divyadṛṣṭiḥ prajāyate //51//

khecari siddhi is obtainedthrough the practice of *neti*. It destroys *kapha doṣas* (disorders of the *kapha*) and *divyadṛṣṭi* (clairvoyance) is attained. -51.

Laulikī

अमन्दवेगेन तुन्दं भ्रामयेदुभपार्श्वयोः ।

सर्वरोगान्निहन्तीह देहानलविवर्धनम् ॥५२॥

amandavegena tundaṃ bhrāmayedubhapārśvayoḥ /

sarvarogānnihantīha dehānalavivarddhanam //52//

Rotate the abdominal muscles very quickly from one side to another. The practice of *Laulikī* destroys all diseases and increases *deha anala* (the bodily fire i.e. digestive fire). -52.

Trāṭaka

निमेषोन्मेषकं त्यक्त्वा सूक्ष्मलक्ष्यं निरीक्षयेत् ।

यावदश्रूणि पतन्ति त्राटकं प्रोच्यते बुधैः ॥५३॥

nimeṣonmeṣam tyaktvā sūkṣmalakṣyam nirīkṣayet /

patanti yāvadaśrūṇi trāṭakum procyate budhaiḥ //53//

Having stopped the blinking of eyes, gaze at a small object until tears shed down. This is called *trāṭaka* by the wise. -53.

एवमभ्यासयोगेन शाम्भवी जायते ध्रुवम् ।

नेत्ररोगा विनश्यन्ति दिव्यदृष्टिः प्रजायते ॥५४॥

evamabhyāsayogena śāmbhavī jāyate dhruvam /

netrarogā vinasyanti divyadṛṣṭiḥ prajāyate //54//

The state of *śāmbhavī mudrā*is attained through this yogic practice. This practice destroys all diseases of the eyes and bestows *divyadṛṣṭi* (clairvoyance). -54.

Kapālabhāti

वातक्रमव्युत्क्रमेण शीत्क्रमेण विशेषतः ।

भालभाति त्रिधा कुर्यात्कफदोषं निवारयेत् ॥५५॥

vātakrameṇa vyutkrameṇa śītkrameṇa viśeṣataḥ /

bhālabhātiṃ tridhā kuryātkaphadoṣaṃ nivārayet //55//

There are three kinds of *kapālabhāti* especially: - *vātakrama*, *vyut-krama* and *śītkrama*. They destroy all disorders arising from *kapha* (phlegm). -55.

Vātakrama

इडया पूरयेद्वायुं रेचयेत्पिङ्गलया पुनः ।

पिङ्गलया पूरयित्वा पुनश्चन्द्रेण रेचयेत् ॥५६॥

iḍayā pūrayedvāyuṃ recayetpiṅgalayā punaḥ /

piṅgalayā pūrayitvā punaścandreṇa recayet //56//

Inhale the air through the left nostril and exhale through the right nostril and again inhale it through the right nostril and exhale it through the left nostril. -56.

पूरकं रेचकं कृत्वा वेगेन न तु धारयेत् ।

एवमभ्यासयोगेन कफदोषं निवारयेत् ॥५७॥

purakaṃ rechakaṃ kṛtvā vegena na tu dhārayet /

evamabhyāsayogena kapha doṣaṃ nivārayet //57//

The inhalation and exhalation should be done without any force. The disorder of the *kapha* (phlegm) is destroyed through this yogic practice. -57.

Vyutkrama

नासाभ्यां जलमाकृष्य पुनर्वक्त्रेण रेचयेत् ।

पायं पायं व्युत्क्रमेण श्लेष्मदोषं निवारयेत् ॥५८॥

nāsābhyāṃ jalamākṛsya punarvaktreṇa recayet /

pāyaṃ pāyaṃ vyutkrameṇa śleṣmādoṣaṃ nivārayet //58//

Draw water through both nostrils and expel it through the mouth, again draw water through the mouth and expel it through the nostrils. In this way, drawing water and expelling it repeatedly destroys the disorder of the *kapha* (phlegm). -58.

Śītkrama

शीत्कृत्य पीत्वा वक्त्रेण नासानलैर्विरेचयेत् ।

एवमभ्यासयोगेन कामदेवसमो भवेत् ॥५९॥

sītkṛtya pītvā vaktreṇa nāsānālairvirecayet /

evamabhyāsayogena kāmadeva samo bhavet //59//

Drink water through the mouth with a hissing sound and expel it through the nostrils. One becomes equal to *kāmadeva* (the God of love) through this yogic practice. -59.

न जायते वार्द्धकं च ज्वरो नैव प्रजायते ।

भवेत्स्वच्छन्ददेहश्च कफदोषं निवारयेत् ॥ ६० ॥

na jāyate vārddhakaṃ ca jvaro naiva prajāyate /

bhavetsvacchanda dehaśca kapaha doṣaṃ nivārayet //60//

One who practices it does not become old and his body does not become frail. The body becomes free (from diseases), healthy and *kapha doṣa* (disorder of phlegm) is removed. -60.

इति श्रीघेरण्डसंहितायां घेरण्डचण्डसंवादे

षड्कर्मशोधनं नाम प्रथमोपदेशः ॥

iti śrīgheraṇḍasamhitāyāṃ gheraṇḍacaṇḍasaṃvāde

ṣaṭkarmasādhanaṃ nāma prathamopadeśaḥ //

Thus ends the First Chapter of *Gheraṇḍa Samhitā*

entitled *Ṣaṭkarma* practice.

Chapter Two

Discourse On Āsana

घेरण्ड उवाच ।

आसनानि समस्तानि यावन्तो जीवजन्तवः ।

चतुरशीतिलक्षाणि शिवेन कथितानि च ॥ १ ॥

gheraṇḍa uvāca /

āsanāni samastāni yāvanto jīvajantavaḥ /

caturaśīti lakṣāṇi śivena kathitāni ca //1//

Sage *Gheraṇḍa* said: - There are as many āsanas as there are living beings in the universe. Lord *Śiva* has described eighty-four hundred thousand āsanas. -1.

तेषां मध्ये विशिष्टानि षोडशोनं शतं कृतम् ।

तेषां मध्ये मर्त्यलोके द्वात्रिंशदासनं शुभम् ॥ २ ॥

teṣāṃ madhye viśiṣṭāni ṣoḍaśonaṃ śataṃ kṛtam/

teṣāṃ madhye martyaloke dvātrimśadāsanaṃ śubham //2//

Of these, eighty-four are the excellent; and of these eighty-four, thirty-two are auspicious in this *martyaloka* (world of mortals). -2.

Kinds of Āsana

सिद्धं पद्मं तथा भद्रं मुक्तं वज्रं च स्वस्तिकम् ।

सिंहं च गोमुखं वीरं धनुरासनमेव च ॥३॥

मृतं गुप्तं तथा मात्स्यं मत्स्येन्द्रासनमेव च ।

गोरक्षं पश्चिमोत्तानमुत्कटं सङ्कटं तथा ॥४॥

मयूरं कुक्कुटं कूर्मं तथा चोत्तानकूर्मकम् ।

उत्तानमण्डूकं वृक्षं मण्डूकं गरुडं वृषम् ॥५॥

शलभं मकरं चोष्ट्रं भुजङ्गं च योगासनम् ।

द्वात्रिंशदासनानि तु मर्त्यलोके हि सिद्धिदम् ॥६॥

siddhaṃ padmaṃ tathā bhadraṃ muktaṃ vajraṃ ca svastikam /
simhaṃ ca gomukhaṃ vīraṃ dhanurāsanameva ca //3//
mṛtaṃ guptaṃ tathā mātsyaṃ matsyendrāsanameva ca /
gorakṣaṃ paścimottānamuṭaṭaṃ saṅkaṭaṃ tathā //4//
mayūraṃ kukkuṭaṃ kūrmaṃ tathā cottānakūrmakam /
uttānamaṇḍukaṃ vṛkṣaṃ maṇḍukaṃ garuḍaṃ vṛṣam //5//
salabhaṃ makaraṃ coṣṭraṃ bhujaṅgaṃ yogamāsanam /
dvātrimśadāsanāni tu martyaloke hi siddhidam //6//

The thirty-two āsanas which certainly bestow *siddhi* (perfection) in this mortal world are: - 1. *siddhāsana*, 2. *padmāsana*, 3. *bhadrāsana*, 4. *muktāsana*, 5. *vajrāsana*, 6. *svastikāsana*, 7. *simhāsana*, 8. *gomukhāsana*, 9. *vīrāsana*, 10. *dhanurāsana*, 11. *mṛtāsana*, 12. *guptāsana*, 13. *mātsyāsana*, 14. *matsyendrāsana*, 15. *gorakṣāsana*, 16. *paścimottānāsana*, 17. *utkaṭāsana*, 18. *saṅkaṭāsana*, 19.

mayūrāsana, 20. *kukkuṭāsana,* 21. *kūrmāsana,* 22. *uttāna kūrmakāsana,* 23. *uttāna maṇḍukāsana,* 24. *vṛkṣāsana,* 25. *maṇḍukāsana,* 26. *garuḍāsana,* 27. *vṛṣāsana,* 28. *salabhāsana,* 29. *makarāsana,* 30. *uṣṭrāsana,* 31. *bhujaṅgāsana* and 32. *yogāsana.* -3-6.

1. Siddhāsana

योनिस्थानकमङ्घ्रिमूलघटितं सम्पीड्य गुल्फेतरं ।

मेढ्रोपर्यथ संनिधाय चिबुकं कृत्वा हृदि स्थापितम् ॥७॥

स्थाणुः संयमितेन्द्रियोऽचलदृशा पश्यन्भ्रुवोरन्तरे ।

एवं मोक्षविधायते फलकरं सिद्धासनं प्रोच्यते ॥८॥

yonisthānakamaṅghrimūlaghaṭitaṃ sampiḍya gulphetaram /

meḍhroparyatha sannidhāya cibukaṃ kṛtvā hṛdi sthāpitam /7/

sthāṇuḥ samyamitendriyo'caladṛśā paśyanbhruvorantaram

hyetanmokṣakapāṭabhedanakaraṃ siddhāsanam procyate /8/

A yogi who has restrained his senses should place one heel at the perineum, theother heel above the penis pressing the pubis and the chin on the chest. Remaining steady and upright, he should fix his gaze constantly between the two eyebrows. This is called *siddhāsana* which breaks open the door to liberation. -7-8.

2. Padmāsana

वामोरूपरि दक्षिणं हि चरणं संस्थाप्य वामं तथा

दक्षोरूपरि पश्चिमेन विधिना कृत्वा कराभ्यां दृढम् ।

अङ्गुष्ठौ हृदये निधाय चिबुकं नासाग्रमालोकयेत्

एतद्व्याधिविकारनाशनकरं पद्मासनं प्रोच्यते ॥९॥

vāmorupari dakṣiṇam hi caraṇam samsthāpya vāmam tathā

dakṣorūpari paścimena vidhinā dhṛtvā karābhyāṃ dṛdham /

aṅguṣṭhau hṛdaye nidhāya cibukaṃ nāsāgramālokayet

etadvyādhivikāranāśanakaraṃ padmāsanaṃ procyate //9//

Place the right foot on the left thigh and the left foot on the right thigh. Then, place the arms behind the back crosswise, firmly grab the big toes and rest the chin on the chest and fix the gaze on the tip of the nose. This is called *padmāsana* which destroys all kinds of diseases. -9.

3. Bhadrāsana

गुल्फौ च वृषणस्याधोव्युत्क्रमेण समाहितः ।

पादाङ्गुष्ठौ कराभ्यां च धृत्वा च पृष्ठदेशतः ॥१०॥

जालन्धरं समासाद्य नासाग्रमवलोकयेत् ।

भद्रासनं भवेदेतत्सर्वव्याधिविनाशाकम् ॥११॥

gulphau ca vṛṣaṇasyādhovyutkrameṇa samāhitaḥ /

pādāṅguṣṭhau karābhyāṃ ca dhṛtvā vai pṛṣṭhadeśataḥ //10//

jālandharaṃ samāsādya nāsāgramavalokayet /

bhadrāsanaṃ bhavedetatsarvavyādhivināśakam //11//

Turn both heels upward and keep them under the scrotum and grasp the big toes behind the back. After performing the *jālandhara Bandha*, gaze on the tip of the nose. This is *bhadrāsana*, the destroyer of all diseases. -10-11.

4. Muktāsana

पायुमूले वामगुल्फं दक्षगुल्फं तथोपरि ।

समकायशिरोग्रीवं मुक्तासनं तु सिद्धिदम् ॥१२॥

pāyumūle vāmagulphaṃ dakṣagulphaṃ tathopari /

samakāyaśirogrīvaṃ muktāsanaṃ tu siddhidam //12//

One should place the left heel at the base of the anus and the right heel above it. The body, head and neck should be kept straight. This is called *muktāsana* which gives perfection. -12.

5. Vajrāsana

जङ्घाभ्यां वज्रवत्कृत्वा गुदपार्श्वे पदावुभौ ।

वज्रासनं भवेदेतद्योगिनां सिद्धिदायकम् ॥१३॥

jaṅghābhyāṃ vajravatkrtvā gudāpārśve padāvubhau /

vajrāsanaṃ bhavedetadyoginām siddhidāyakam //13//

Making the thighs solid like thunderbolt, the legs are placed by the side of the anus. This is *vajrāsana* which gives perfection to yogis. -13.

6. Svastikāsana

जानूर्वोरन्तरे कृत्वा योगी पादतले उभे ।

ऋजुकायसमासीनः स्वस्तिकं तत्प्रचक्षते ॥१४॥

jānūrvorantare krtvā yogī pādatale ubhe /

rjukāyasamāsīnaḥ svastikam tatpracakṣate //14//

Placing the soles of both feet between the calves and thighs, sit with the body straight and remain stable. That is called *svastikāsana*. -14.

7. Simhāsana

गुल्फौ च वृषणस्याधो व्युत्क्रमेणोर्ध्वतां गतौ ।

चितियुग्मं भूमिसंस्थं करौ च जानुनोपरि ॥१५।

व्यात्तवक्त्र जलन्ध्रेण नासाग्रमवलोकयेत् ।

सिंहासनं भवेदेतत्सर्वव्याधिविनाशकम् ॥१६॥

gulphau ca vṛṣaṇasyādho vyutkrameṇordhvatāṃ gatau /

citiyugmaṃ bhūmisamsthaṃ karau ca jānunopari //15//

vyāttavaktro jalandhreṇa nāsāgramavalokayet /

simhāsanaṃ bhavedetatsarvavyādhivināśakam //16//

Place both the heels under the scrotum with the feet crosswise turning upward. Place the knees on the ground and hands on them with open mouth. Then, practice *jālandhara bandha* and fix the gaze on the tip of the nose. This is called *simhāsana*, the destroyer of all diseases. -15-16.

8. Gomukhāsana

पादौ च भूमौ संस्थाप्य पृष्ठपार्श्वे निवेशयेत् ।

स्थिरं कायं समासाद्य गोमुखं गोमुखाकृतिः ॥१७॥

pādau ca bhūmau samsthāpya pṛṣṭhapārśve niveśayet /

sthiraṃ kāyaṃ samāsādhya gomukhaṃ gomukhākṛtiḥ //17//

Place both feet on the ground with the heels crosswise on each side of the buttocks. Sit calmly keeping the body stable with the mouth raised. This is *gomukhāsana* forming the shape of the mouth of a cow. -17.

9. Vīrāsana

एकं पादमथैकस्मिन्विन्यसेदूरुसंस्थितम् ।

इतरस्मिस्तथा पश्चाद्वीरासनमितीरितम् ॥१८॥

ekaṃ pādamathaikasminvinyasedūrusamsthitam /

itarasminstathā paścādvīrāsanamitīritam //18//

Place the right foot near the thigh of left foot. Then bend the left knee and turn the foot backwards. This is called *vīrāsana.* -18.

10. Dhanurāsana

प्रसार्य पादौ भुवि दण्डरूपौ

करौ च पृष्ठे धृतपादयुग्मम् ।

कृत्वा धनुस्तुल्यपरिवर्तिताङ्गं

निगद्यते वै धनुरासनं तत् ॥१९॥

prasārya pādau bhuvi daṇḍarūpau

   karau ca pṛṣṭhe dhṛtapādayugmam /

kṛtvā dhanurvatparivartitāṅgaṃ

   nigadhyate vai dhanurāsanam tat //19//

Lie down facing on the ground and extend both legs like a stick. Then grab both ankles with hands and stretch the body making it like a bow. This is called *dhanurāsana*. -19.

11. Mṛtāsana

उत्तानं शववद्भूमौ शायानं तु शवासनम् ।

शवासनं श्रमहरं चित्तविश्रान्तिकारणम् ॥२०॥

uttānaṃ śavavatbhūmau śayanaṃ tu śavāsanam /

savāsanaṃ śramaharaṃ cittaviśrāntikārakam //19//

Lying down on the ground like a dead person is *śavāsana*. *Śavāsana* removes fatigue and relaxes the mind. -20.

12. Guptāsana

जानूर्वोरन्तरे पादौ कृत्वा पादौ च गोपयेत् ।

पादोपरि च संस्थाप्य गुदं गुप्तासनं विदुः ॥२१॥

jānūrvorantare pādau kṛtvā pādau ca gopayet /

pādopari ca samsthāpya gudaṃ guptāsanam viduḥ //21//

Keep both feet in the middle of the knees and thighs, and place the anus area between the feet. This is called *guptāsana*. -21.

13. Matyāsana

मुक्तपद्मासनं कृत्वा उत्तानशयनं चरेत् ।

कूर्पराभ्यां शिरो वेष्ट्यं रोगघ्नं मत्स्यासनम् ॥२२॥

muktapadmāsanaṃ kṛtvā uttānaśayanaṃ caret /

kūrparābhyāṃ śiro veṣṭyaṃ rogaghnaṃ mātsyamāsanam //22//

After performing *muktapadmāsana*, lie flat on the ground resting the head between the two elbowsof the hands. This is called *mātsyāsana*, the destroyer of diseases. -22.

14. Matsyendrāsana

उदरं पश्चिमाभासं कृत्वा तिष्ठत्ययत्नतः ।

नम्रितं वामपादं हि दक्षजानूपरि न्यसेत् ॥२३॥

तत्र याम्यं कूर्परं च याम्यकरेऽपि च।

भ्रुवोर्मध्ये गतां दृष्टिः पीठं मात्स्येन्द्रमुच्यते ॥२४॥

udaraṃ paścimābhāsaṃ kṛtvā tiṣṭhatyayatnataḥ /

namritaṃ vāmapādaṃ hi dakṣajānūpari nyaset //23//

tatra yāmyaṃ kūrparaṃ ca yāmyakare 'pi ca /

bhruvormadhye gatāṃ dṛṣṭiḥ pīṭhaṃ mātsyendramucyate //24//

After pulling the abdomen backward, remain upright with due effort. Bend the left leg and place the heel/foot on the right thigh. Place the right elbow on the leg, the chin on the right hand and fix the gaze between the eyebrow center. This is called *matsyendrāsana*. -23-24.

15. Gorakṣāsana

जानूर्वोरन्तरे पादौ उत्तानौ व्यक्तसंस्थितौ ।

गुल्फौ चाच्छाद्य हस्ताभ्यामुत्तानाभ्यां प्रयत्नतः ॥२५॥

कण्ठसङ्कोचनं कृत्वा नासाग्रमवलोकयेत् ।

गोरक्षासनमित्याहुर्योगिनां सिद्धिकारणम् ॥२६॥

jānūrvorantare pādau uttānau vyaktasaṃsthitau /

gulphau cācchādya hastābyāmuttānābhyāṃ prayatnataḥ //25//

kaṇṭhasaṅkocanaṃ kṛtvā nāsāgramavalokayet /

gorakṣāsanamityāhuryogināṃ siddhikārakam //26//

Keep the both feet turned upward concealed in the middle of the knees and the thighs, and then cover the heels carefully with both the hands turned upward. After contracting the throat, fix the gaze at the tip of the nose. This is called *gorakṣāsana* which gives perfection to yogis. -25-26.

16. Paścimottānāsana

प्रसार्य पादौ भुवि दण्डरूपौ

विन्यस्तभालं चितियुग्ममध्ये ।

यत्नेन पादौ च धृतौ कराभ्यां

तत्पश्चिमोत्तानमिहासनं स्यात् ॥२७॥

prasārya pādau bhuvi daṇḍarūpau

vinyastabhālaṃ citiyugmamadhye /

yatnena pādau ca dhṛtau karābhyāṃ

tatpaścimottānamihāsanaṃ syāt //27//

Stretch both legs out on the ground like a stick and place the forehead between the knees and then grasp the big toes carefully with the hands. This is *paścimottānāsana.* -27.

17. Utkaṭāsana

अङ्गुष्ठभ्यामवष्टभ्य धरां गुल्फौ च खे गतौ ।

तत्रोपरि गुदं न्यस्य विज्ञेयं तुत्कटासनम् ॥२८॥

aṅguṣṭhābhyāmavaṣṭabhya dharāṃ gulphau ca khe gatau /

tatropari gudaṃ nyasya vijñeyaṃ tūtkaṭāsanam // 28//

Keep the big toes on the ground with the heels raised up in the air and place the area of the anus on the heels. This is known as *utkaṭāsana.* -28.

18. Saṅkaṭāsana

वामपादचितेर्मूलं विन्यस्य धरणीतले ।

पाद दण्डेन याम्येन वेष्टयेद्वामपादकम् ।

जानुयुग्मे करयुग्ममेतत्सङ्कटमासनम् ॥२९॥

vāmapādacitermūlaṃ vinyasya dharaṇītale /

pāda daṇḍenayāmyena veṣṭayedvāmapādakam /

jānuyugme karayugmetatsaṅkaṭāsanam //29//

Keeping the left shin and foot on the ground, wrap the right leg around the left leg and then place both the hands on the knees. This is called *saṅkaṭāsana.* -29.

19. Mayūrāsana

पाण्योस्तलामाभ्यामवलम्ब्य भूमिं

तत्कूर्परस्थापितनाभिपार्श्वम् ।

उच्चासनो दण्डवदुत्थित: खे

मायूरमेतत्प्रवदन्ति पीठम् ॥३०॥

pāṇyostalābhyāmavalambya bhūmiṃ

taṭūrparasthāpitanābhipārśvam /

uccāsano daṇḍavadutthitaḥ khe

māyūrametatpravadanti pīṭham //30//

Placing the palms of both hands firmly on the floor, keep both elbows on each side of the navel region. Then raise both legs and the body like a stick in the air. This is called *mayūrāsana*. -30.

20. Kukkuṭāsana

पद्मासनं समासाद्य जानूर्वोरन्तरे करौ ।

कूर्पराभ्यां समासीनो उच्चस्थः कुक्कुटासनम् ॥३१॥

padmāsanaṃ samāsādhya jānūrvorantare karau /

kūrparābhyāṃ samāsīno uccasthaḥ kukkuṭāsanam //31//

Sitting in *padmāsana*, insert the hands between the thighs and calves. Place the palms firmly on the floor and raise the body with the support of the elbows. This is called *kukkuṭāsana*. -31.

21. Kūrmāsana

गुल्फौ च वृषणस्याधो व्युत्क्रमेण समाहितौ ।

ऋजुकायशिरोग्रीवं कूर्मासनमितीरितम् ॥३२॥

gulphau ca vṛṣaṇasyādho vyutkrameṇa samāhitau /

ṛjukāyaśirogrīvaṃ kūrmāsanamitīritam //32//

Place both heels under the scrotum/testes opposite to one another and keep the body, head and neck straight. This is called *kūrmāsana*. -32.

22. Uttāna Kūrmāsana

कुक्कुटासनबन्धस्थं कराभ्यां धृतकन्धरम् ।

पीठं कूर्मवदुत्तानमेतदुत्तानकूर्मकम् ॥३३॥

kukkuṭāsanabandhastham karābhyām dhṛtakandharam /

pīṭham kūrmavaduttānametaduttānakūrmakam //33//

Perform *kukkuṭāsana*, then hold the shoulders with the hands and straighten the body like a tortoise. This is *uttānakūrmāsana*. -33.

23. Maṇḍukāsana

पृष्ठदेशे पादतलावङ्गुष्ठौ द्वौ च संस्पृशेत् ।

जानुयुग्मं पुरस्कृत्य साधयेन्मण्डूकासनम् ॥३४॥

pṛṣṭhadeśe pādatalāvaṅguṣṭhau dvau ca saṃspṛśet /

jānuyugmam puraskṛtya sādhyenmaṇḍūkāsanam //34//

Bring both feet behind the back and join the big toes keeping the knees apart in front. Thus, *maṇḍūkāsana* is practiced. -34.

24. Uttāna Maṇḍūkāsana

मण्डूकासनमध्यस्थं कूर्पराभ्यां धृतं शिरः ।

एतद्भेकवदुत्तानमेतदुत्तानमण्डूकम् ॥३५॥

maṇḍūkāsanamadhyastham kūrparābhyām dṛtam śiraḥ /

etadbhekavaduttānametaduttānamaṇḍukam //35//

Performing *maṇḍūkāsana*, the head is held on the elbows lifting up the torso like a frog. This is *uttānamaṇḍukāsana*. -35.

25. Vṛkṣāsana

वामोरुमूलदेशे च याम्यं पादं निधाय तु ।

तिष्ठेत्तु वृक्षवद्भूमौ वृक्षासनमिदं विदुः ॥३६॥

vāmorumūladeśe ca yāmyaṃ pādaṃ nidhāya vai /

tiṣṭhettu vṛkṣavatbhūmau vṛkṣāsanamidaṃ viduḥ//36//

Placing the right foot at the root of the left thigh, stand straight on the ground like a tree. This is called *vṛkṣāsana.* -36.

26. Garuḍāsana

जङ्घोरुभ्यां धरां पीड्य स्थिरकायो द्विजानुना ।

जानूपरि करद्वन्द्वं गरुडासनमुच्यते ॥३७॥

jaṅghorubhyāṃ dharāṃ pīḍya sthirakāyo dvijānunā /

jānūpari karadvandvaṃ garuḍāsanamucyate //37//

Pressing the ground firmly with both the thighs and knees, keep the body stable and place both hands on the knees. This is called *garuḍāsana.* -37.

27. Vṛṣāsana

याम्यगुल्फे पायुमूले वामभागे पदेतरम् ।

विपरीतं स्पृशेद्भूमिं वृषासनमिदं भवेत् ॥३८॥

yāmyagulphe pādamūle vāmabhāge padetaram /

viparītaṃ spṛśedbhūmim vṛṣāsanamidaṃ bhavet //38//

Placing the anus on the right heel, bring the left heel on the left side of the anus and keep the left foot on the ground facing backwards. This is called the *vṛṣāsana.* -38.

28. Śalabhāsana

अध्यास्य शेते करयुग्मवक्ष

आलम्ब्य भूमिं करयोस्तलाभ्याम् ।

पादौ च शून्ये च वितस्ति चोर्ध्वं

वदन्ति पीठं शलभं मुनीन्द्राः ॥३९॥

adhyāsya śete karayugmavakṣa

    ālambya bhumiṃ karayostalābhyām /

pādau ca śūnye ca vitasti cordhyaṃ

    vadanti pīṭhaṃ śalabhaṃ munīndrāḥ //39//

Lie down facing on the ground. Keep both arms by the sides of the chest placing the palms firmly on the ground and raise both legs in the air. This is called *śalabhāsana* by the great sages. 39.

29. Makarāsana

अध्यास्य शेते हृदयं निधाय

भूमौ च पादौ च प्रसार्यमाणौ ।

शिरश्च धृत्वा करदण्डयुग्मे

देहाग्निकारं मकरासनं तत् ॥४०॥

adyāsya śete hṛdayaṃ nidhāya

    bhūmau ca pādau prasāryamāṇau /

śirasca dhṛtvā karadaṇḍayugme

    dehāgnikāraṃ makarāsanam tat //40//

Lie down facing on the ground with the chest touching the floor. Spread out the legs and hold the head on the arms. This is *makarāsana* which activates the bodily fire. -40.

30. Uṣṭrāsana

अध्यास्य शेते पदयुग्मव्यस्तं

पृष्ठे निधायापि धृतं कराभ्याम् ।

आकुञ्च्य सम्यग्ध्युदरास्यगाढं

उष्ट्रं च पीठं यतयो वदन्ति ॥४१॥

adhyāsya śete padayugmavyastaṃ

  pṛṣṭhe nidhāyāpi dhṛtaṃ karābhyām/

ākuñcya samyagdhyudarāsyagāḍhaṃ

  uṣṭraṃ ca pīṭhaṃ yatayo vadanti //41//

Lie down facing on the ground. Bending both legs, cross them behind the back. Holding the feet with the hands, contract the mouth and the abdomen forcefully. This is called *uṣṭrāsana* by the ascetics. -41.

31. Bhujaṅgāsana

अङ्गुष्ठनाभिपर्यन्तमधोभूमौ विनिन्यसेत् ।

  धरां करतलाभ्यां धृत्वोर्ध्वशीर्ष फणीव हि ॥४२॥

देहाग्निर्वर्धते नित्यं सर्वरोगविनाशनम् ।

  जागर्ति भुजङ्गीदेवी भूजङ्गासनसाधनात् ॥४३॥

aṅguṣṭhanābhiparyantamadhobhūmau ca vinyaset /

dharāṃ karatalābhyāṃ dhṛtvordhvaśīrṣam phaṇīva hi //42//

dehāgnivarddhate nityaṃ sarvarogavināśanam /

jāgarti bhujaṅgīdevī bhujaṅgāsanasādhanāt //43//

Place the body facing down from the toes to the navel on the floor. Placing the palms of the hands firmly on the floor, raise the head like a snake. This is *bhujaṅgāsana* which increases the fire of the body and destroys all diseases. *Bhujaṅgīdevī* (i.e. the divine serpent power) is awakened by the practice of this asana. -42-43.

32. Yogāsana

उत्तानौ चरणौ कृत्वा संस्थाप्योपरि जानुनो: ।

आसनोपरि संस्थाप्य चोत्तानं करयुग्मकम् ॥४४॥

पूरकैर्वायुमाकृष्य नासाग्रमवलोकयेत् ।

योगासनं भवेदेतद्योगिनां योगसाधने ॥४५॥

uttānau caraṇau kṛtvā saṃsthāpyopari jānunoḥ /

āsanopari saṃsthāpya cottānaṃ karayugmakam //44//

pūrakairvāyumākṛṣya nāsāgramavalokayet /

yogāsanaṃ bhavedetadyogināṃ yogasādhane //45//

Turning the feet upwards, place them on the opposite knees. Keep both hands on the knees with the palm turned upwards. Inhale, hold the air inside and fix the gaze at the tip of the nose. This is *yogāsana* which should be practiced by the yogis. -44-45.

इति श्रीघेरण्डसंहितायां घेरण्डचण्डकापालिसंवादे

आसनप्रयोगो नाम द्वितीयोपदेशः ॥

iti śrīgheraṇḍasamhitāyāṃ gheraṇḍacaṇḍasaṃvāde

āsanaprayogo nāma dvitīyopadeśaḥ /

Thus ends the Second Chapter of *Gheraṇḍa Samhitā* entitled Āsana Practice.

Chapter Three

Discourse On Mudrā

Types of Mudrās

घेरण्ड उवाच ।

महामुद्रा नभोमुद्रा उड्डीयानं जलन्धरम् ।

मूलबन्धं महाबन्धं महावेधश्च खेचरी ॥ १ ॥

विपरीतकरी योनिर्वज्रोणी शक्तिचालनी ।

ताडागी माण्डुकी मुद्रा शाम्भवी पञ्चधारणा ॥ २ ॥

अश्विनी पाशिनी काकी मातङ्गी च भुजङ्गिनी ।

पञ्चविंशतिमुद्राश्च सिद्धिदा इह योगिनाम् ॥ ३ ॥

gheraṇḍa uvāca /

mahāmudrā nabhomudrā uḍḍīyānaṃ jalandharam /

mūlabandho mahābandho mahāvedhaśca khecarī //1//

viparītakarī yonirvajroṇi śakticalanī /

tāḍāgī māṇḍukī mudrā śāmbhavī pañcadhāraṇā //2//

aśvinī pāśinī kākī mātaṅgī ca bhujaṅginī /

pañcavimśatimudrāśca siddhidā iha yoginām //3//

Sage *Gheraṇḍa* said: - *Mahā mudrā, nabho mudrā, uḍḍīyāna bandha, jālandhara bandha, mūla bandha, mahā bandha, mahā bedha mudrā, khecarī mudrā, viparīta karani mudrā, yoni mudrā, vajroṇi mudrā, śakti cālinī mudrā, tāḍāgī mudrā, māṇḍukī mudrā, śāmbhavī mudrā, pañcadhāraṇās* (the five concentrations), *aśvinī mudrā, pāśinī mudrā, kākī mudrā, mātaṅginīmudrā* and *bhujaṅginī mudrā* are the twenty-five *mudrās* which give *siddhi* (perfection) to yogis. -1-3.

मुद्राणां पटलं देवि कथितं तव संनिधौ ।

येन विज्ञातमात्रेण सर्व सिद्धिः प्रजायते ॥४॥

गोपनीयं प्रयत्नेन न देयं यस्यकस्यचित् ।

प्रीतिदं योगिनां चैव दुर्लभं मरुतामपि ॥५॥

mudrāṇām paṭalam devi kathitam tava sannidhau /

yena vijñātamātreṇa sarva siddhiḥ prajāyate //4//

gopanīya prayatnena na deyam yasyakasyacit /

prītidam yoginām caiva durlabhamarutāmapi //5//

Mahesvara talking to *Devi* about *mudrās* said: - O *Devi*! I have told you about the chapter dealing with the *mudrās*. Through their knowledge alone leads to all perfection/mastery in yoga. This knowledge of the *mudrās* should be kept secret with due effort. It should not be imparted to everyone. Their knowledge gives bliss to yogis which is not easily available even to the Gods. -4-5.

1. Mahāmudrā

पायुमूलं वामगुल्फे संपीड्य दृढयत्नतः ।

याम्यपादं प्रसार्याथ करोपात्तपदाङ्गुलः ॥६॥

कण्ठसङ्कोचनं कृत्वा भ्रुवोर्मध्यं निरीक्षयेत् ।

महामुद्राभिधा मुद्रा कथ्यते चैव सूरभिः ॥७॥

क्षयकासं गुदावर्तप्लीहाजीर्णज्वरं तथा ।

नाशयेत्सर्वरोगांश्च महामुद्रा च साधनात् ॥८॥

pāyumūlaṃ vāmagulphe sampīḍya dṛḍhayatnataḥ /

yāmyapādaṃ prasāryātha karopāttapadāṅgulaḥ //6//

kaṇṭhaṃ saṅkocanaṃ kṛtvā bhruvormadhyaṃ nirīkṣayet /

mahāmudrābhidhā mudrā kathyate caiva sūrabhiḥ //7//

kṣayakāsaṃ gudāvartaplīhājīrṇajvaraṃ tathā /

nāsayetsarvarogāmśca mahāmudrā ca sādhanāt //8//

Pressing the anus area with the left heel carefully, stretch the right leg in front and take hold of the toes with both hands. After contracting the throat, focus the gaze in the middle of the eyebrow center. This is called *mahā mudrā* by the wise. The practice of *mahā mudrā* cures tuberculosis, disorders of phlegm, constipation, enlarged spleen and fever. Through the practice/mastery of *mahā mudrā* all diseases are cured. -6-8.

2. Nabho Mudrā

यत्र यत्र स्थितो योगी सर्वकार्येषु सर्वदा ।

ऊर्ध्वजिह्वः स्थिरो भूत्वा धारयेत्पवनं सदा ।

नभोमुद्रा भवेदेषा योगिनां रोगनाशिनी ॥९॥

yatra yatra sthito yogī sarvakāryeṣu sarvadā /

urdhvajihvaḥ sthiro bhūtvā dhārayetpavanaṃ sadā /

nabhomudrā bhavedeṣā yogināṃ roganāśinī //9//

Wherever a yogi is and whatever activity he is engaged in, he should steadily turn the tongue upwards and always retain the breath. This is *nabho mudrā* which destroys all the diseases of the yogi. -9.

3. Uḍḍiyāna Bandha

उदरे पश्चिमं तानं नाभेरूर्ध्वं तु कारयेत् ।

उड्डीनं कुरुते यस्मादविश्रान्तं महाखगः ।

उड्डीयान त्वसौ बन्धो मृत्युमातङ्गकेसरी ॥१०॥

समग्राद् बन्धनाध्येतदुड्डीयानं विशिष्यते ।

उड्डीयाने समभ्यस्ते मुक्तिः स्वाभाविकी भवेत् ॥११॥

udare paścimaṃ tānaṃ nābhirūrdhvaṃ tu kārayet /

uḍḍīnaṃ kurute yasmādaviśrāntaṃ mahākhagaḥ /

uḍḍīyānaṃ tvasau bandho mṛtumātaṅgakesarī //10//

samagrād bandhanāddhyetaduḍḍīyānaṃ viśiṣyate /

uḍḍīyāne samabhyste muktiḥ svābhāvikī bhavet //11//

Contract the abdomen equally above the navel towards the back. Consequently, the great dynamic bird (*prāna*) flies upward. This is called *uḍḍīyāna bandha*. It is a victorious lion over the elephant of death. Of all the *bandhas, Uḍḍīyāna bandha* is the chief one. Liberation is accomplished naturally through its proper practice. -10-11.

4. Jālandhara Bandha

कण्ठसङ्कोचनं कृत्वा चिबुकं हृदये न्यसेत् ।

जालन्धरेकृते बन्धे षोडशाधारबन्धनम् ।

जालन्धरमहामुद्रा मृत्योश्च क्षयकारिणी ॥ १२ ॥

सिद्धो जालन्धरो बन्धो योगिनां सिद्धिदायक: ।

षण्मासमभ्यसेद्यो हि स सिद्धो नात्र संशयः ॥ १३ ॥

kaṇṭhasaṅkocanaṃ kṛtvā cibukaṃ hṛdaye nyaset /

jālandharekṛte bandhe ṣoḍaśādhārabandhanam //12//

jālandharamahāmudrā mṛtyośca kṣayakāriṇī /

siddho jālandharo bandho yogināṃ siddhidāyakaḥ /

ṣaṇmāsamabhyasedyo hi sa siddho nātra saṃśayaḥ //13//

While contracting the throat, place the chin on the chest. This is the practice of *jalandhara bandha*. The sixteen *ādhāras* (bases or supports) are controlled by this practice. This great *mudrā* named *jālandhara bandha* destroys death. Mastery over *jālandhara bandha* bestows *siddhis* to yogis. A yogi certainly becomes a *siddha* (perfected one) by just practicing it for six months. There is no doubt about it. - 12-13.

5. Mūlabandha

पार्ष्णिना वामपादस्य योनिमाकुञ्च्चयेत्ततः ।

नाभिग्रन्थि मेरुदण्डे सुधीः संपीड्य यत्नतः ॥ १४ ॥

मेढ्रं दक्षिणगुल्फेन दृढबन्धं समाचरेत् ।

नाभेरूर्ध्वमधश्चापि तानं कुर्यात्प्रयत्नतः ।

जराविनाशिनी मुद्रा मूलबन्धो निगद्यते ॥ १५ ॥

संसारसागरं तर्तुमभिलषति यः पुमान् ।

सुगुप्तो विरलो भूत्वा मुद्रामेतां समभ्यसेत् ॥ १६ ॥

अभ्यासाद्बन्धनस्यास्य मरुत्सिद्धिर्भवेद्ध्रुवम् ।

साधयेद्यत्नतस्तर्हि मौनी तु विजितालसः ॥१७॥

pārṣṇinā vāmapādasya yonimākuñcayettataḥ /

nābhigranthiṃ merudaṇḍe sudhiḥ sampīḍya yatnataḥ //14//

meḍhram dakṣiṇagulphena dṛḍhabandhaṃ samācaret /

jarāvināśinī mudrā mūlabandho nigadhyate //15//

saṃsārasāgaraṃ tartumabhilaṣati yaḥ pumān /

sugupto viralo bhūtvā mudrāmetāṃ samabhyaset //16//

abhyāsādbandhanasyāsya marutsiddhirbhaveddhruvam /

sādhayedyatnatastarhi mauni tu vijitālasaḥ //17//

Pressing the genital area between the anus and testes with the left heel, contract the anus. Press the navel knot close to the spinal column with due effort and firmly press the genital organ with the right heel. This is called *mūla bandha* which destroys old age. The wise yogis who wish to cross the ocean of the world should practice this *mudrā* in a secret and solitary place. *Maruta siddhi* (perfection of *prāna* or *vāyu*) is certainly attained through this practice. Therefore, one should practice it with due effort in silence without laziness. -14-17.

6. Mahābandha

वामपादस्य गुल्फेन पायुमूलं निरोधयेत् ।

दक्षपादेन तद्गुल्फं संपीड्य यत्नतः सुधीः ॥१८॥

शनैः शनैश्चालयेत्पार्ष्णिं योनिमाकुञ्चयेच्छनैः ।

जालन्धरे धरेत्राणं महाबन्धो निगद्यते ॥१९॥

महाबन्धः परो बन्धो जरामरण नाशनः ।

प्रसादादस्य बन्धस्य साधयेत्सर्ववाञ्छितम् ॥२०॥

vāmapādasya gulphena pāyumūlaṃ nirodhayet /

dakṣapādena tadgulpham sampīḍya yatnataḥ sudhīḥ //18//

śanaiḥ sanaiścālayetpārṣṇi yonimākuñcayecchanaiḥ /

jālandhare dharetprāṇaṃ mahābandho nigadyate //19//

mahābandhaḥ paro bandho jarāmaraṇa nāśanaḥ /

prasādādasya bandhasya sādhayetsarvavāñchitam //20//

Closing the anus with the left heel, press the left heel with the right foot with due effort. Slowly contract and expand the perineum and retain the breath by applying *jālandhara bandha*. This is called *mahā bandha*. It is the supreme *bandha* (of all the *bandhas*) and is the destroyer of old age and death. All desires objects are accomplished through the grace of this *bandha*. -18-20.

7. Mahāvedha Mudrā

रूपयौवनलावण्यं नारीणां पुरुषं विना ।

मूलबन्धमहाबन्धौ महावेधं विना तथा ॥२१॥

महाबन्धं समासाद्य कुम्भकं चरेत्दुड़ीन।

महावेधः समाख्यातो योगिनां सिद्धिदायकः ॥२२॥

महाबन्धमूलबन्धौ महावेधसमन्वितौ ।

प्रत्यहं कुरुते यस्तु स योगी योगवित्तमः ॥२३॥

न मृत्युतो भयं तस्य न जरा तस्य विद्यते ।

गोपनीयः प्रयत्नेन वेधोऽयं योगिपुङ्गवैः ॥२४॥

rūpayauvanalāvaṇyaṃ nārīṇām puruṣam vinā /

mūlabandhamahābandhau mahāvedhaṃ vinā tathā //21//

mahābandhaṃ samāsādya kumbhakaṃ careduḍḍīna /

mahāvedaḥ samākhyāto yoginām siddhidāyakaḥ //22//

mahābandhamūlabandhau mahāvedasamanvitau /

pratyahaṃ kurute yastu say yogī yogavittamaḥ //23//

na mṛtyuto bhayaṃ tasya na jarā tasya vidyate /

gopanīyaḥ prayatnena vedho 'yaṃ yogipuṅgavaiḥ //24//

As the beauty, youth and charisma of a woman are worthless without a man, similarly are the *mūla bandha* and *mahā bandha* without *mahā veda*. First perform *mahā bandha* and then while doing *uḍḍīyāna bandha* retain the breath by *kumbhaka*. This is called *mahā veda*, the giver of *siddhis* to all yogis. The yogi who practice *mahā bandha* and *mūla bandha* daily along with *mahā veda*, becomes the best of all yogis. There is no fear of old age and death for him. The wise yogi should carefully keep this *vedha* secret. -21-24.

8. Khecarī Mudrā

जिह्वाधो नाडीं सञ्छित्य रसनां चालयेत्सदा ।

दोहयेन्नवनीतेन लौहयन्त्रेण कर्षयेत् ॥२५॥

एवं नित्यं समभ्यासाल्लम्बिका दीर्घतां व्रजेत् ।

यावद्गच्छेद्भ्रुवोर्मध्ये तदा सिध्यति खेचरी ॥२६॥

रसनां तालुमूले तु शनैः शनैः प्रवेशयेत् ।

कपालकुहरे जिह्वा प्रविष्टा विपरीतगा ।

भ्रुवोर्मध्ये गता दृष्टिर्मुद्रा भवति खेचरी ॥२७॥

jihvādho nāḍīṃ sañchitya rasanām cālayetsadā /

dohayennavanītena lauhayantreṇa karṣayet //25//

evaṃ nityaṃ samabhyāsāllambika dīrghatāṃ vrajet /

yāvadgacchedbhruvormadhye tadā sidhyati khecari //26//

rasanāṃ tālumūle tu śanaiḥ śanaiḥ praveśayet /

kapālakuhare jihvā praviṣṭā viparītagā /

bhruvormadhye gatā dṛṣṭirmudrā bhavati khecari //27//

Cutting the tendon (frenulum) at the base of the tongue, move the tongue constantly. Rub it with fresh butter and milk it out slowly with a pair of iron forceps. In this way, the tongue is elongated through proper regular practice. When the tongue reaches the eyebrow center, then *khecari mudrā* is accomplished. Thus, insert the tongue into the base of the palate slowly and gently. Turning the tongue upwards and backwards, take and enter the tongue into the holes of the nasal passage. Keep the gaze fixed at the eyebrow center. This becomes *khecari mudrā*. -25-27.

न च मूर्च्छा क्षुधा तृष्णा नैवालस्यं प्रजायते ।

न च रोगो जरा मृत्युर्देवदेहः स जायते ॥२८॥

नाग्निना दह्यते गात्रं न शोषयति मारुतः ।

न देहं क्लेदयन्त्यापो दशेन्न भुजङ्गमः ॥२९॥

लावण्यं च भवेद्गात्रे समाधिर्जायते ध्रुवम् ।

कपालवक्त्रसंयोगे रसना रसमाप्नुयात् ॥३०॥

na ca mūcchā kṣudhā tṛṣṇā naivālasyaṃ prajāyate /

na ca rogo jarā mṛtyurdevadehaḥ sa jāyate //28//

nāgninā dahyate gātraṃ na śoṣayati mārutaḥ /

na dehaṃ cledayantyāpo daśenna bhujaṅgamaḥ //29//

lāvaṇyaṃ ca bhavedgātre samādhirjāyate dhruvaṃ /

kapālavaktrasamyoge rasanā rasamāpnuyāt //30//

Through the practice of *khecari mudrā* neither there is faint nor hunger, nor thirst, nor laziness. Neither there is disease, nor old age, nor death. The body becomes divine. The physical body is neither burnt by fire, nor dried up by air, nor it is made wet by water, nor it is affected by the poison of snake bite. The body becomes beautiful. *Samādhi* is certainly accomplished. Various juices are obtained through the union of the tongue between the forehead and mouth. -28-30.

नानारससमुद्भूतमानन्दं च दिने दिने ।

आदौ च लवणं क्षारं च ततस्तिक्तकषायकम् ॥३१॥

नवनीतं घृतं क्षीरं दधितक्रमधूनि च ।

द्राक्षारसं च पीयूषं जायते रसनोदकम् ॥३२॥

nānārasasamudbhūtamānandaṃ ca dine dine /

ādau ca lavaṇaṃ kṣāraṃ ca tatastiktakaṣāyakam //31//

nanītaṃ gṛtaṃ kṣīraṃ dadhitakramadhūni ca /

drākṣārasaṃ ca pīyūsaṃ jāyate rasanodakam //32//

Various types of juices are produced every day and a blissful state is experienced. At first salty and alkaline, then bitter and astringent tastes are felt and then taste of butter, ghee, milk, yogurt, buttermilk, honey, grape juice are felt and finally, the taste of nectar arises. -31-32.

9. Viparīrakaraṇī Mudarā

नाभिमूले वसेत्सूर्यस्तालुमूले च चन्द्रमाः ।

अमृतं ग्रसते सूर्यस्ततो मृत्युवशो नरः ॥३३॥

ऊर्ध्वं च योजयेत्सूर्यं चन्द्रं चाप्यध आनयेत् ।

विपरीतकरी मुद्रा सर्वतन्त्रेषु गोपिता ॥३४॥

भूमौ शिरश्च संस्थाप्य करयुग्मं समाहितः ।

ऊर्ध्वपादः स्थिरो भूत्वा विपरीतकरी मता ॥३५॥

मुद्रां च साधयेन्नित्यं जरा मृत्युं च नाशयेत् ।

स सिद्धः सर्वलोकेषु प्रलयेऽपि न सीदति ॥३६॥

nābhimūle vasetsūryastālumūle ca candramāḥ /

amṛtaṃ grasate sūryastato mṛtyuvaśo naraḥ //33//

urdhvaṃ ca yojayetsūryaṃ candraṃ cāpyadha ānayet /

viparītakarī mudrā sarvatantreṣu gopitā //34//

bhūmau śiraśca samsthāpya karayugmaṃ samāhitaḥ /

urdhvapādaḥ sthiro bhūtvā viparītakarī matā // 35//

mudrā ca sādhayennityaṃ jarā mṛtu ca nāśayet /

sa siddhaḥ sarvalokeṣu pralaye'pi na sīdati //36//

The sun (i.e. the solar plexus) is situated at the root of the navel and the moon is situated at the root of the palate. A man is subject to death because the sun devours the nectar. Hence, the sun should be brought upward and the moon downward. This is *viparītakaraṇī mudrā* which is kept secret in all the *tantras*. Placing the head on the ground, support with both hands spreading out. Raise both legs and remain stable. This is *viparītakaraṇī mudrā*. By daily practice of this *mudrā* one destroys old age and death. He becomes an adept in all the worlds and does not suffer even at the time of dissolution. -33-36.

10. Yoni Mudrā

सिद्धासनं समासाद्य कर्णचक्षुर्नसामुखम् ।

अङ्गुष्ठतर्जनी मध्यानामादिभिश्च धारयेत् ॥३७॥

काकीभिः प्राणसङ्कृष्य अपाने योजयेत्ततः ।

षड्ऋकाणि क्रमाध्यात्वा हुं हंसमनुना सुधीः ॥३८॥

चैतन्यमानयेद्देवीं निद्रिता या भुजङ्गिनी ।

जीवेन सहितां शक्तिं समुत्थाप्य पराम्बुजे ॥३९॥

शक्तिमयः स्वयं भूत्वा परं शिवेन सङ्गमम् ।

नानासुखं विहारं च चिन्तयेत्परमं सुखम् ॥४०।

शिवशक्तिसमायोगादेकान्तं भुवि भावयेत् ।

आनन्दमानसो स्वयं भूत्वा अहं ब्रह्मेति सम्भवेत् ॥४१॥

योनिमुद्रा परा गोप्या देवानामपि दुर्लभा ।

सकृत्तु लाभसंसिद्धिः समाधिस्थः स एव हि ॥४२॥

siddhāsanaṃ samāsādya karṇacakṣurnasāmukham/

aṅguṣṭha madhyanāmādibhścḁ dhārayet // 37//

kākībhiḥ prāṇasaṅkṛṣya apāne yojayettataḥ /

ṣaṭcakrāṇi kramātdhyātvā hum haṃsamanunā sudhiḥ //38//

caitanyamānayeddevīṃ nidritā yā bhujaṅginī /

jīvena sahitāṃ śaktiṃ samutthāpya parāmbuje //39//

śaktimayaḥ svayaṃ bhutvā paraṃ śivena saṅgamam /

nānāsukhaṃ vihāraṃ ca cintayetparamam sukham //40//

śivaśaktisamāyogādekāntaṃ bhuvi bhāvayet /

ānandamānaso svayaṃ bhūtvā ahaṃ brahmeti sambhavet //41//

yonimudrā parā gopyā devānāmapi durlabhā /

sakṛttu lābhasamsiddhiḥ samādhisthaḥ sa eva hi //42//

Sitting in *siddhāsana*, close the ears with both thumbs, the eyes with the index fingers, both nostrils with the middle fingers and mouth with the ring fingers and the little fingers. Pull the *prāṇa* through *kākīmudrā* and join it with the *apāna*. Meditating on the six *cakras* according to their order, awaken the sleeping *kuṇḍalinī śakti* through the practice of the *mantras* 'hūm' and 'haṃsa'. Raise the *Śakti* along with the individual soul and bring it to *sahasrāra* (the thousand petalled lotus). Being one full of *Śakti* and united with supreme *Śiva* feel that "I am roaming with *Śiva* with all the happiness and I am augmented by *Śakti* and enjoying a blissful state". Contemplate absolutely on the union of *Śiva* and *Śakti* in this world. Being oneself blissful through their union, realize oneself that "I am also *Brahman*". This *yoni mudrā* is highly secret. It is rare even for the Gods. He who accomplishes perfection in it through regular practice, naturally attains the state of *samādhi.* -37-42.

ब्रह्महा भ्रूणहा चैव सुरापी गुरुतल्पगः ।

एतैः पापैर्न लिप्यते योनिमुद्रानिबन्धनात् ॥४३॥

यानि पापानि घोराणि उपपापानि यानि च ।

तानि सर्वाणि नश्यन्ति योनिमुद्रानिबन्धनात् ।

तस्मादभ्यासनं कुर्याद्यादि मुक्ति समिच्छति ॥४४॥

brahmahā bhrūṇahā caiva surāpi gurutalpagaḥ /

etaiḥ pāpairna lipyate yonimudrā nibandhanāt //43//

yāni pāpāni ghoraṇi upapāpāni yāni ca /

tāni sarvāṇi nasyanti yonimudrā nibandhanāt /

tasmādabhyāsanaṃ kuryādyādi muktiṃ samicchati //44//

By the practice this *mudrā* one gets rid of sins like killing a *brāhmaṇa* or a fetus, drinking alcohol or violating the bed of the teacher. All types of great sins and small sins are eradicated by the practice of *yoni mudrā*. Therefore, one should practice it if he sincerely wishes for liberation. -43-44.

11. Vajroṇi Mudrā

धरामवष्टभ्य करयोस्तलाभ्याम्

उर्ध्वे क्षिपेत्पादयुगं शिरः खे ।

शक्तिप्रबोधाय चिरजीवनाय

वज्रोणिमुद्रा मुनयो वदन्ति ॥४५॥

अयं योगे योग श्रेष्ठो योगिनां मुक्तिकारणम् ।

अयं हितप्रदो योगो योगिनां सिद्धिदायकः ॥४६॥

एतद्योगप्रसादेन बिन्दुसिद्धिर्भवेद्धुवम् ।

सिद्धे बिन्दौ महायत्ने किं न सिध्यति भूतले ॥४७॥

भोगेन महता युक्तो यदि मुद्रां समाचरेत् ।

तथापि सकला सिद्धिर्भवति तस्य निश्चितम् ॥४८॥

dharāmavaṣṭabhya karayostalābhyāṃ

urdve kṣipetpādayugaṃ śiraḥ khe /

śaktiprabodhāya cirajīvanāya

vajroṇimudrā munayoḥ vadanti //45//

ayaṃ yoge yoga śreṣṭho yogināṃ muktikāraṇam /

ayaṃ hitaprado yogo yogināṃ siddhidāyakaḥ //46//

etadyogaprasādena bindusiddhirbhaveddhruvam /

siddhe vindu mahāyatne kiṃ na sidhyati bhūtale //47//

bhogena mahatā yukto yadi mudrāṃ samācaret /

tathāpi sakalā siddhirbhavati tasya niścitam //48//

Placing both palms firmly on the ground, raise both legs and the head in the air. The *munis* (seers) have called it *vajroṇi mudrā* which awakens the *Śakti* and provides long life. Due to the grace of this yogic *mudrā*, *bindu siddhi* (perfection in the retention of seminal fluid) is certainly accomplished. When *bindu siddhi* is attained with the highest effort, what cannot be achieved in this world? Even though engaged in great enjoyments, one can certainly attain all the *siddhis* through the perfection of this *mudrā.* -45-48.

12. Śakticālinī Mudrā

मूलाधारे आत्मशक्तिः कुण्डली पर देवता ।

शयिता भुजगाकारा सार्ध त्रिवलयान्विता ॥४९॥

यावत्सा निद्रिता देहे तावज्जीवः पशुर्यथा ।

ज्ञानं न जायते तावत्कोटियोगं समभ्यसेत् ॥५०॥

mūlādhāre ātmaśaktiḥ kuṇḍalī para devatā /

śayitā bhujagākārā sārdha trivalayānvitā //49//

yāvatsā nidritā dehe tāvajjīvaḥ paśuryathā /

jñānaṃ na jāyate tāvat kotiyogaṃ samabhyaset //50//

The supreme goddess *kuṇḍalinī*, the power of the Self, sleeps in *mūlādhāra* in the form of a serpent coiled in three and a half rounds. As long as she is asleep, *jīva* (a living being) remains in ignorance like an animal. Until then the knowledge does not arise even though one may practice ten million types of yoga. -49-50.

उद्धाटयेत्कवाटं च यथा कुञ्चिकया हठात् ।

कुण्डलिन्याः प्रबोधेन ब्रह्मद्वारं प्रभेदयेत् ॥५१॥

नाभिं संवेष्ट्य वस्त्रेण न च नग्नो बहिः स्थितः ।

गोपनीयगृहे स्थित्वा शक्तिचालनमभ्यसेत् ॥५२॥

udghāṭayeṭavātaṃ ca yathā kuñcikayā haṭhāt /

kuṇḍalinyāḥ prabodhena brahmadvāraṃ prabhedayet //51//

nābhiṃ samveṣṭya vastreṇa na ca nagno bahiḥ sthitaḥ /

gopanīyagṛhe sthitvā śakticālanamabhyset //52//

Just like a door is opened after opening the lock with a key, in the same way *brahmadvāra* (the door to *Brahma*) is opened forcibly when *kuṇḍalinī* is awakened. *Śakticālana* should be practiced in a solitary shelter/home covering the navel with a piece of cloth wrapped around (the waist/loins). It should not be practiced being naked in an open area (staying outside). -51-52.

वितस्तिप्रमितं दीर्घं विस्तारे चतुरङ्गुलम् ।

मृदुलं धवलं सूक्ष्मं वेष्टनाम्बरलक्षणम् ।

एवमम्बरयुक्तं च कटिसूत्रेण योजयेत् ॥५३॥

भस्मना गात्रं संलिप्य सिद्धासनं समाचरेत् ।

नासाभ्यां प्राणमाकृष्य अपाने योजयेद्बलात् ॥५४॥

तावदाकुञ्चयेद्गुह्यं शनैरश्विनिमुद्रया ।

यावद्गच्छेत्सुषुम्णायां वायुः प्रकाशयेद्धठात् ॥५५॥

तदा वायुप्रबन्धेन कुम्भिका च भुजङ्गिनी ।

बद्धश्वासस्ततो भूत्वा ऊर्ध्वमार्गं प्रपद्यते ॥५६॥

vitastipramitaṃ dīrghaṃ vistāre caturaṅgulam /

mṛdulam dhavalaṃ sūkṣmaṃ veṣṭanāmbaralakṣaṇam /

evamambarayuktaṃ ca katisūtreṇa yojayet //53//

bhasmanā gātraṃ samlipya siddhāsanaṃ samācaret /

nāsābhyāṃ prāṇamākṛṣya apāne yojayetbalāt //54//

tāvadākuñcayedguhyaṃ śanairaśvinimudrayā /

yāvadgacchetsuṣumṇāyāṃ vāyuḥ prakāśayeddhaṭhāt //55//

tadā vāyuprabandhena kumbhikā ca bhujaṅginī /

baddhaśvāsastato bhūtvā ūrdvāmārgaṃ prapadhyate //56//

The wrapping cloth should be soft, white and fine measuring about 10 centimeters wide and 23 centimeters long. Fasten this cloth around the navel with a *katisūtra* (a cotton thread/rope which is worn around the loins). Smearing the ashes on the whole body, sit in *siddhāsana*. Drawing the *prāṇa* inside, join it by force with the *apāna*. Contract the anus slowly by practicing *aśvini mudrā* until the *prāṇa* passes through the *suṣumṇā* and manifests forcibly there. Thus, with the *prāṇa* held by *kumbhaka,* the *kuṇḍalinī* in the form of serpent being suffocated awakens and then follows the upward passage. – 53-56.

विना शक्तिचालनेन योनिमुद्रा न सिध्यति ।

आदौ चालनमभ्यस्य योनिमुद्रां समभ्यसेत् ॥५७॥

इति ते कथितं चण्डकापाले शक्तिचालनम् ।

गोपनीयं प्रयत्नेन दिने दिने समभ्यसेत् ॥५८॥

vinā śakticālena yonimudrā na sidhyati /

ādau cālanamabhasya yonimudrāṃ samabhyaset //57//

iti te kathitaṃ caṇḍakāpāle śakticālanam /

gopanīya prayatnena dine dine samabhyaset //58//

Without the practice of *śakticālana mudrā, yoni mudrā* cannot be accomplished. First one should practice *śakticālana* properly and then duly practice *yoni mudrā.* O *Caṇḍakapāli!* Thus, I have told you about *śakticālana mudrā.* Keeping it secret with care, practice it daily. -57-58.

मुद्रेयं परमा गोप्या जरामरणनाशिनी ।

तस्मादभ्यसनं कार्यं योगिभिः सिद्धिकाङ्क्षिभिः ॥५९॥

नित्यं योऽभ्यसते योगी सिद्धिस्तस्य करे स्थिता ।

तस्य विग्रहसिद्धिः स्याद्रोगाणां सङ्क्षयो भवेत् ॥६०॥

mudreyam paramā gopyā jaramaraṇanaśinī /

tasmādabhyasanaṃ kāryam yogibhih siddhikāṅkṣibhih //59//

nityaṃ yo 'bhyasate yogī siddhistasya kare sthitā /

tasya vigrahasiddhih syādrogāṇāṃ saṅkṣayo bhavet //60//

This *mudrā* is highly secret. It destroys old age and death. Therefore, the yogis and those who are desirous of *siddhis* (perfections) should do its practice. The yogi who practices it daily, the *siddhis* dwell in his hand. He attains *vigraha siddhi* (perfection of the body) and all his diseases are eliminated entirely. -59-60.

13. Taḍāgi Mudrā

उदरं पश्चिमोत्तानं कृत्वा च तडागाकृति ।

ताडागी सा परामुद्रा जरा मृत्यु विनाशिनी ॥६१॥

udaraṃ paścimottānam kṛtvā ca taḍāgākṛtih /

tāḍāgi sā parāmudrā jarā mṛtyu vināśinī //61//

Sitting in *paścimottānāsana*, enlarge the abdomen fully like a shape of a pond. This is *tāḍāgi,* a great *mudrā* which destroys old age and death. -61.

14. Māṇḍukī Mudrā

मुखं समुद्रितं कृत्वा जिह्वामूलं प्रचालयेत् ।

शनैर्ग्रसेदमृतं तां माण्डुकीं मुद्रिकां विदुः ॥६२॥

वलितं पलितं नैव जायते नित्ययौवनम् ।

न केशो जायते पाको यः कुर्यान्नित्यमाण्डुकीम् ॥६३॥

mukhaṃ samudritaṃ kṛtvā jihvāmūlaṃ pracālayet /

śanairgrasedamṛtaṃ tāṃ māṇḍukīṃ mudrikāṃ viduḥ //62//

valitaṃ palitaṃ naiva jāyate nityayauvanam /

na keśe jāyate pāko yaḥ kuryānnityamāṇḍukīm //63//

Keeping the mouth closed, rotate the tongue inside the palate and taste the nectar slowly by the tongue. This is called *māṇḍukīmudrā*. By the practice of this *mudrā* regularly wrinkles and grey hairs never appear in the body. Long-lasting youth is attained. -62-63.

15. Śāmbhavī Mudrā

नेत्राञ्जनं समालोक्य आत्मारामं निरीक्षयेत् ।

सा भवेच्छाम्भवी मुद्रा सर्वतन्त्रेषु गोपिता ॥६४॥

अथ शाम्भवीमुद्रायाः फलकथनम् ।

वेदशास्त्रपुराणानि सामान्यगणिका इव ।

इयं तु शाम्भवीमुद्रा गुप्ता कुलवधूरिव ॥६५॥

स एव आदिनाथश्च स च नारायणः स्वयम् ।

स च ब्रह्मा सृष्टिकारी यो मुद्रां वेत्ति शाम्भवीम् ॥६६॥

netrāñjanaṃ samālokya ātmārāmaṃ nirīkṣayet /

sā bhavetcchāmbhavī mudrā sarvatantreṣu gopitā //64//

vedaśāstrapurāṇāni sāmānyagaṇikā iva /

iyaṃ tu śāmbhavīmudrā guptā kulavadhūriva //65//

sa eva ādināthaśca sa ca nārāyaṇaḥ svayam /

sa ca brahmā sṛṣṭikārī yo mudrāṃ vetti śāmbhavīm //66//

Fix the gaze steadily between the eyebrows, observe the Self within. This is *śāmbhavī mudrā* which is kept secret in all the *tantras*. The *Vedas, Śāstras* and *Purāṇas* are like ordinary women, but *śāmbhavī mudrā* is like a lady of a noble family. One who knows *śāmbhavī mudrā* is himself *Ādinātha, Nārāyaṇa* and *Brahmā*, the creator of the world. -64-66.

सत्यं सत्यं पुनः सत्यं सत्यमुक्तं महेश्वरः ।

शाम्भवीं यो विजानीयात्स च ब्रह्म न चान्यथा ॥६७॥

satyaṃ satyaṃ punaḥ satyaṃ satyamuktaṃ maheśvaraḥ /

śāmbhavīṃ yo vijānīyātsa ca brahma na cānyathā //67//

Maheśvara says: - "It is true, it is true and it is verily true again that he who knows *śāmbhavī mudrā* is certainly *Brahma*. There is no doubt about it." -67.

Pañcadhāraṇā

कथिता शाम्भवी मुद्रा श्रृणुष्व पञ्चधारणाम् ।

धारणानि समासाद्य किं न सिध्यति भूतले ॥६८॥

अनेन नरदेहेन स्वर्गेषु गमनागमम् ।

मनोगतिर्भवेत्तस्य खेचरत्वं न चान्यथा ॥६९॥

kathitā śāmbhavimudrā śruṇusva pañcadhāraṇām /

dhāraṇāni samāsādya kiṃ na sidhyati bhūtale //68//

anena naradehena svargeṣu gamanāgamam /

manogatirbhavettasya khecaratvaṃ na cānyathā //69//

Śāmbhavī mudrā has been explained above. Now listen to *pañca dhāraṇā* (the five concentrations which are *pārthivī, āmbhasī, āgneyī, vāyavīya* and *ākāśī*). After having mastery over them, what cannot be

[60]

accomplished in this universe? With this human body one can travel to heaven and come back to earth. By these *dharanas* one acquires *manogati* (the power to go anywhere at one's will with the speed of mind) and *khecaratva* (the ability to travel in space). -68-69.

16. Pārthivī Dhāraṇā

यत्तत्वं हरितालदेशरचितं भौमं लकाराऽन्वितं

वेदास्त्रं कमलासनेन सहितं कृत्वा हृदिस्थायिनम् ।

प्राणस्तत्र विलीय पञ्चघटिकाश्चित्तान्वितां धारयेत्

एषा स्तम्भकरी सदा क्षितिजयं कुर्यादधोधारणा ॥७०॥

पार्थिवीधारणामुद्रां यः करोति तु नित्यशः ।

मृत्युञ्जयः स्वयं सोऽपि स सिद्धो विचरेद्भुवि ॥७१॥

yattvaṃ haritāladeśaracitaṃ bhaumaṃ lakārānvitaṃ

vedāstraṃ kamalāsanenasahitaṃ kṛtvā hṛdisthāpitam /

prāṇastatra vilīya pañcaghaṭikāścittānvitāṃ dhārayet

eṣā stambhakarī sadā kṣitijayaṃ kuryādadhodhāraṇā //70//

pārthivīdhāraṇāmudrāṃ yaḥ karoti tu nityaśaḥ /

mṛtuñjayaḥ svayaṃ so'pi sa siddho vicaredbhuvi //71//

The earth element has yellow color, the *bīja mantra* relating to it is '*lam*', it has a square shape and its god in lotus pose is *Brahmā*. Establish this *tattva* in the heart, dissolve the *prāṇa* thereby *kumbhaka* and focus the mind on it for five *ghaṭikās* (two hours). This is called *adhodhāraṇā*. By perfecting this practice one always acquires steadiness and conquers the earth. One who practises *prithvidhāraṇā* daily conquers death himself. He becomes a *siddha* (perfected one) and roams on this earth. -70-71.

17. Āmbhasī Dhāraṇā

शाङ्ख्रेन्दुप्रतिमं च कुन्दधवलं तत्त्वं किलालं शुभं

तत्पीयूषवकारबीजसहितं युक्तं सदा विष्णुना ।

प्राणं तत्र विलीय पञ्चघटिकाश्चित्तान्वितां धारयेत्

एषा दुःसहतापपापहरिणी स्यादाम्भसी धारणा ॥७२॥

śaṅkhendupratimaṃ ca kundadhavalaṃ

tattvaṃ kilālaṃ śubhaṃ /

tatpīyūṣavakārbījasahitaṃ yuktaṃ sadā viṣṇunā /

prāṇaṃ tatra vilīya pañcaghaṭikāścitānvitāṃ dhārayet /

eṣā duḥsahatāpapāpahariṇī syādāmbhasī dharaṇā //72//

The water element has white color which is like the color of a jasmine flower or a conch or the moon. It has a circular shape and the *bīja mantra* of this ambrosial element is '*vam*'. It is always associated with Lord *Viṣṇu*. Focus on this element in the heart and dissolve the *prāṇa* there through *kumbhaka* practice for five *ghaṭikās* (two hours). This is *āmbhasī dhāraṇā* which destroys pains, sufferings and sins all together. -72.

आम्भसीं परमां मुद्रां यो जानाति स योगवित् ।

जले च घोरे गंभिरे मरणं तस्य नो भवेत् ॥७३॥

इयं तु परमा मुद्रा गोपनीया प्रयत्नतः ।

प्रकाशात्सिद्धिहानिः स्यात्सत्यं वच्मि च तत्त्वतः ॥७४॥

āmbhāsīṃ paramāṃ mudrāṃ yo jānāti sa yogavit /

jale ca ghore gambhīre maraṇaṃ tasya no bhavet //73//

iyaṃ tu paramā mudrā gopanīyā prayatnataḥ /

prakāśātsiddhihāniḥ syātsatyaṃ vacmi ca tattvataḥ //74//

Āmbhasī is a supreme *mudrā*. One who knows it is the knower of yoga. A person never dies even in very deep water through the practice of this *mudrā*. Keep this supreme *mudrā* carefully secret. The *siddhi* is destroyed by disclosing it. Surely, I have told you the truth. -73-74.

18. Āgneyī Dhāraṇā

यन्नाभिस्थितमिन्द्रगोपसदृशं बीजं त्रिकोणान्वितं

तत्त्वं वह्निमयं प्रदीप्तमरुणं रुद्रेण यत्सिद्धिदम् ।

प्राणं तत्र विलीय पञ्चघटिकाश्चित्तान्वितं धारयेत्

एषा कालगभीरभीतिहरणी वैश्वानरी धारणा ॥७५॥

yannābhisthitamindragopasadṛśam bījaṃ trikoṇānvitam,

tattvaṃ vahnimayaṃ pradīptamaruṇam rudreṇa yatsiddhidam /

prāṇam tatra vilīya pañcaghaṭikāścittānvitaṃ dhārayet,

eṣā kālagabhīrabhītihariṇī vaisvānarī dhāraṇā //75//

The fire element is located at the navel region. Its color is red like the cochineal insect. It has a triangular shape. Its *bīja mantra* is 'ram' and it deity is *Rudra*. This element is full of flaming fire and has the radiance of the sun. It is the giver of *siddhi* (perfection). Contemplating on this element, dissolve the *prāṇa* there for five *ghaṭikās* (two hours). This is *vaisvānarī dhāraṇā* which destroys the fear of horrible death. -75.

प्रदीप्ते ज्वलिते वह्नौ यदि पतति साधकः ।

एतन्मुद्राप्रसादेन स जीवति न मृत्युभाक् ॥७६॥

pradīpte jvalite vahnau patito yadi sādhakaḥ /

etanmudrā prasādena sa jīvati na mṛtyubhāk //76//

If a *sādhaka* falls into a flaming fire, he remains alive and does not face the jaws of death by the grace of this *mudrā*. -76.

19. Vāyavīya Dhāraṇā

यद्भिन्नाञ्जनपुञ्जसंनिभमिदं धूम्राऽवभासं परं,

तत्त्वं सत्त्वमयं यकारसहितं यत्रेश्वरो देवता ।

प्राणं तत्र विलीय पञ्चघटिकाश्चित्तान्वितं धारयेत्

एषा खे गमनं करोति यामिनां स्याद्वायवी धारणा ॥७७॥

yadbhinnāñjanapuñjasannibhamidaṃ

    dhūmrāvabhāsaṃ param,

tattvaṃ sattvamayam yakārasahitaṃ yatreśvaro devatā /

prāṇaṃ tatra vilīya pañcaghatikāścittānvitaṃ dhārayet,

eṣā khe gamanaṃ karoti yāmināṃ syādvāyavī dhāraṇā //77//

The color of the air element is black like collyrium or smoke. Its *bīja mantra* is 'yam'. This *tattva* is full of *sāttvika* qualities and its *devatā* (god/deity) is *Iśvara*. Focus on this element in the heart and dissolve the *prāṇa* there by *kumbhaka* practice with concentrated mind for five *ghaṭikās* (two hours). This is *vāyavī dhāraṇā*. The practitioner travels in space by the practice of this *mudrā*. -77.

इयं तु परमा मुद्रा जरामृत्युविनाशिनी ।

वायुनाम्रियते नापि खे च गतिप्रदायिनी ॥७८॥

शठाय भक्तिहीनाय न देयं यस्यकस्यचित् ।

दत्ते च सिद्धिहानिः स्यात्सत्यं वच्मि च चण्ड ते ॥७९॥

iyaṃ tu paramā mudrā jarāmṛtyuvināśinī /

vāyunāmriyate nāpi khe ca gatipradāyinī //78//

śaṭhāya bhaktihīnāya na deyaṃ yasyakasyacit /

datte ca siddhihāniḥ syātsatyaṃ vacmi ca caṇḍe te //79//

This is a foremost *mudrā* which destroys decay and death. One cannot be killed because of air and gains the power to fly in space. This *dhāraṇā* should never be taught to those who are wicked and devoid of devotion. If it is given, *siddhi* is verily destroyed. O *Caṇḍakapāli!* Surely, I have told you the truth. -78-79.

20. Ākāśī Dhāraṇā

यत्सिन्धौ वरशुद्धवारिसदृशं व्योमाख्यमुद्धासते

तत्त्वं देवसदाशिवेन सहितं बीजं हकारान्वितम् ।

प्राणं तत्र विलीय पञ्चघटिकाश्चित्तान्वितं धारयेद्

एषा मोक्षकवाटभेदनकरी कुर्यान्नभोधारणा ॥८०॥

yatsindhau varaśuddhavārisadṛśaṃ vyomākhyamudbhāsate,

tattvaṃ devasadāśivena sahitaṃ bījaṃ hakārānvitam /

prāṇaṃ tatra vilīya pañcaghaṭikāścittānvitaṃ dhārayet,

eṣā mokṣakapāṭabhedanakarī kuryānnabhodhāraṇā //80//

The eather element has the colour of pure ocean water. Its *bīja mantra* is 'haṃ' and its deity is *Sadāśiva*. Dissolve the *prāṇa* by *kumbhaka* practice with concentrated mind there for five *ghaṭikās* (two hours). This is *nabho dhāraṇā mudrā* which opens the gate to liberation. It should be practiced. -80.

आकाशीधारणां मुद्रां यो वेत्ति स च योगवित् ।

न मृत्युर्जायते तस्य प्रलये नावसीदति ॥८१॥

ākāśīdhāraṇāṃ mudrāṃ yo vetti sa yogavit /

na mṛtyurjāyate tasya pralaye nāvasīdati //81//

One who knows *ākāśī dhāraṇā mudrā* is the knower of yoga. He does not die even at the time of dissolution. – 81.

21. Aśvinī Mudrā

आकुञ्चयेद्गुदद्वारं प्रकाशयेत् पुनः पुनः ।

सा भवेदश्विनी मुद्रा शक्तिप्रबोधकारिणी ॥८२॥

अश्विनी परमा मुद्रा गुह्यरोगविनाशिनी ।

बलपुष्टिकरी चैव अकालमरणं हरेत् ॥८३॥

ākuñcayed gudadvāraṃ prakāśayet punaḥ punaḥ /

sā bhavedaśvinīmudrā śaktiprabodhakāriṇī //82//

aśvinī paramā mudrā guhyarogavināśinī /

balapuṣṭikarī caiva akālamaraṇam haret //83//

Contract and expand the anus area repeatedly. It is called *aśvinī mudrā*. It awakens the *kuṇḍalinī śakti*. This is a foremost *mudrā* which destroys all hidden diseases (i.e. anus, rectum and reproductive organs). It provides physical strength and nourishment, and prevents untimely death. -82-83.

22. Pāśinī Mudrā

कण्ठपृष्ठे क्षिपेत्पादौ पाशवद् दृढबन्धनम् ।

सा एव पाशिनी मुद्रा शक्तिप्रबोधकारिणी ॥८४॥

पाशिनी महती मुद्रा बलपुष्टिविधायिनी ।

साधनीया प्रयत्नेन साधकैः सिद्धिकाङ्क्षिभिः ॥८५॥

kaṇṭhapṛṣṭhe kṣipetpādau pāśavad dṛḍhabandhanam /

sā eva pāśinī mudrā śaktiprabodhakāriṇī //84//

paśinī mahatī mudrā balapuṣṭividhāyinī /

sādhaniyā prayatnena sādhakaiḥ siddhikāṅkṣibhiḥ //85//

Cast both legs behind the neck and tie up them firmly like a noose. This is called *pāśinī mudrā*. It awakens the *kuṇḍalinī śakti*. *Pāśinī* is a great *mudrā* which gives strength and nourishment. A *sādhaka* desirous of *siddhi* should practice it with due effort. -84-85.

23. Kākī Mudrā

काकचञ्चुवदास्येन पिबेद्वायुं शनैः शनैः ।

काकी मुद्रा भवेदेषा सर्वरोगविनाशिनी ॥८६॥

काकीमुद्रा परा मुद्रा सर्वतन्त्रेषु गोपिता ।

अस्याः प्रसादमात्रेण काकवन्निरुजो भवेत् ॥८७॥

kākacañcuvadāsyena pibedvāyuṃ śanaiḥ śanaiḥ /

kākī mudrā bhvedeṣā sarvarogavināśinī //86//

kākīmudrā parā mudrā sarvatantreṣu gopitā /

asyāḥ prasādamātreṇa kākavannīrujo bhavet //87//

Inhale slowly through the mouth making its shape like a beak of a crow. This is *kākī mudrā*, the destroyer of all diseases. This is an important *mudrā* kept secret in all the *tantras*. By the grace of this *mudrā*, one becomes free from diseases like a crow. -86-87.

24. Mātaṅginī Mudrā

कण्ठमग्नेजले स्थित्वा नासाभ्यां जलमाहरेत् ।

मुखान्निर्गमयेत्पश्चात् पुनर्वक्त्रेण चाहरेत् ॥८८॥

नासाभ्यां रेचयेत्पश्चात् कुर्यादेवं पुनः पुनः ।

मातङ्गिनी परा मुद्रा जरामृत्यु विनाशिनी ॥८९॥

kaṇṭhamagnejale sthitvā nāsābhyāṃ jalamāharet /

mukhānnirgamayetpaścāt punarvaktreṇa cāharet //88//

nāsābhyāṃ recayetpaścāt kuryādevaṃ punaḥ punaḥ /

mātaṅginī parā mudrā jarāmṛtyu vināśinī //89//

Stand in water up to the neck level deep. Inhale drawing the water up through the nostrils and expel it out through the mouth. Then draw the water through the mouth and expel it through the nostrils. This practice should be repeated. This is a great *mātaṅginī mudrā* which destroys old age and death. -88-89.

विरले निर्जने देशे स्थित्वा चैकाग्रमानसः ।

कुर्यान्मातङ्गिनीं मुद्रां मातङ्ग इव जायते ॥९०॥

यत्र यत्र स्थितो योगी सुखमत्यन्तमश्नुते ।

तस्मात्सर्वप्रयत्नेन साधयेत् मुन्द्रिकां पराम् ॥९१॥

virale nirjane deśe sthitvā caikāgramānasaḥ /

kuryānmātaṅginī mudrāṃ mātaṅga iva jāyate //90//

yatra yatra sthito yogī sukhamatyantamaśnute /

tasmātsarvaprayatnena sādhayet mudrikāṃ parām //91//

A yogi should practice it remaining alone in an isolated place with a concentrated mind. By this *mudrā* he becomes strong like an elephant. Wherever he stays, he remains in a great happiness. Therefore, this great *mudrā* should be perfected with the highest effort. -90-91.

25. Bhujaṅginī Mudrā

वक्त्रं किञ्चित्सुप्रसार्य चाऽनिलं गलया पिबेत् ।

सा भवेद्भुजङ्गी मुद्रा जरामृत्युविनाशिनी ॥९२॥

यावच्च उदरे रोगमजीर्णादि विशेषतः ।

तत्सर्वं नाशयेदाशु यत्र मुद्रा भुजङ्गिनी ॥९३॥

vaktraṃ kiñcitsuprasārya cānilaṃ galayā pibet /

sā bhavedbhujaṅgī mudrā jarāmṛtyuvināśinī //92//

yāvacca udare rogamajīrṇādi viśeṣataḥ /

tatsarvaṃ nāśayedāśu yatra mudrā bhujaṅginī //93//

Opening the mouth a little wide, draw air through the throat. This becomes *bhujaṅginī mudrā*, the destroyer of old age and death. All digestive disorders, especially indigestion, etc. are destroyed at once by the mastery over this *mudrā*. -92-93.

Fruits of the Mudras

इदं तु मुद्रापटलं कथितं चण्डकापाले ।

वल्लभं सर्वसिद्धानां जरामरणनाशनम् ॥९४॥

शठाय भक्तिहीनाय न देयं यस्य कस्यचित् ।

गोपनीयं प्रयत्नेन दुर्लभं मरुतामपि ॥९५॥

ऋजवे शान्तचित्ताय गुरुभक्तिपराय च ।

कुलीनाय प्रदातव्यं भोगमुक्ति प्रदायकम् ॥९६॥

idaṃ tu mudrāpaṭalaṃ kathitaṃ caṇḍakāpāle /

vallabham sarvasiddhānāṃ jarāmaraṇanāsanam //94//

śaṭhāya bhaktihīnāya na deyaṃ yasya kasyacit /

gopaniyaṃ prayatnena durlabham marutāmapi //95//

ṛjave śāntacittāya gurubhakti parāya ca /

kulīnāya pradātavyaṃ bhogamukti pradāyakam //96//

Now the benefits of the *mudrās* are described.

O *Caṇḍakapāli!* Here I have told you the chapter on *mudrās*. They are dear to all *siddhas*. They destroy old age and death. Do not teach them to people who are wicked and devoid of devotion. Keep them secret carefully as they are rare even to gods. These *mudrās* should be taught to those who are mentally peaceful, devoted to their gurus and who belong to a noble family. These *mudrās* provide both worldly enjoyments and liberation. -94-96.

मुद्राणां पटलं ह्येतत्सर्वव्याधिविनाशनम् ।

नित्यमभ्यासशीलस्य जठराग्निविवर्धनम् ॥९७॥

न तस्य जायते मृत्युर्नास्य जरादिकं तथा ।

नाग्निजलभयं तस्य वायोरपि कुतो भयम् ॥९८॥

कासः श्वासः प्लीहा कुष्ठं श्लेष्मरोगाश्च विंशतिः ।

मुद्राणां साधनाच्चैव विनश्यन्ति न संशयः ॥९९॥

mudrāṇāṃ paṭalaṃ hyetatsarvavyādhi vināśanam /

nityamabhyāsa śīlasya jaṭharāgnivivardhanam //97//

na tasya jāyate mṛtyurnāsya jarādikaṃ tathā /

nāgnijalabhayaṃ tasya vāyorapi kuto bhayam //98//

kāsaḥ śvāsaḥ plihā kuṣṭhaṃ śleṣmarogāśca vimśatiḥ //

mudrāṇāṃ sadhanāccaiva vinasyanti na samśayaḥ //99//

All diseases are destroyed by these *mudrās* explained in this chapter. The digestive fire of a *sādhaka* is activated through their regular practice. He is not touched by death and old age. He has no fear of fire, water and air. Twenty types of diseases like cough, asthma, spleen disorders, leprosy and phlegm, etc., are destroyed through the practice of these *mudrās*. There is no doubt about it. -97-99.

बहुना किमिहोक्तेन सारं वच्मि च चण्ड ते ।

नास्ति मुद्रासमं किञ्चित्सिद्धिदं क्षितिमण्डले ॥१००॥

bahunā kimihoktena sāraṃ vacmi ca caṇḍa te /

nāsti mudrāsamaṃ kiñcitsiddhidam kṣitimaṇḍale //100//

O *Caṇḍakapāli!* What shall I tell you more? I have explained you in summary. There is nothing equal to these *mudrās* for granting *siddhis* in this world. -100.

इति श्रीघेरण्डसंहितायां घेरण्डचण्डसंवादे

मुद्राप्रयोगो नाम तृतीयोपदेशः ॥

iti śrīgheraṇḍasamhitāyāṃ gheraṇḍacaṇḍasamvāde

mudrāprayogo nāma tṛtīyopadeśaḥ /

Thus ends the Third Chapter of *Gheraṇḍa Samhitā* entitled *Mudrā* Practice.

Chapter Four

Discourse On Pratyāhāra

घेरण्ड उवाच ।

अथातः सम्प्रवक्ष्यामि प्रत्याहारकमुत्तमम् ।

यस्य विज्ञानमात्रेण कामादिरिपुनाशनम् ॥१॥

gheraṇḍa uvāca /

athātaḥ sampravakṣyāmi pratyāhārakamuttamam /

yasya vijñānamātreṇa kāmādiripunāśanam //1//

Sage *Gheraṇḍa* said: - Now I shall describe you the highest practice of *pratyāhāra*. By knowing this alone, all the enemies like *kāmā* (craving, lust), etc. are destroyed. -1.

यतो यतो निश्चरति मनश्चञ्चलमस्थिरम् ।

ततस्ततो नियम्यैतदात्मन्येव वशं नयेत् ॥२॥

yato yato niścarati manaścañcalamasthiram /

tatastato niyamyaitadātmanyeva vaśaṃ nayet //2//

Whenever the mind wanders and become unstable, subduing it, bring it back under control of *Ātma* (the Self). -2.

पुरस्कारं तिरस्कारं सुश्राव्यं वा भयानकम् ।

मनस्तस्मान्नियम्यैतदात्मन्येव वशं नयेत् ॥३॥

puraskāraṃ tiraskāraṃ suśrāvyaṃ vā bhayānakam /

manastamānniyamyaitadātmanyeva vaśam nayet //3//

Respect or condemnation, hearing of good words or very bad words, subdue the mind in all these (contradictions) and bring it back under control of *Ātma* (the Self). -3.

सुगन्धे वाऽपि दुर्गन्धे मनो घ्राणेषु जायते ।

तस्मात्प्रत्याहरेदेतदात्मन्येव वशं नयेत् ॥४॥

sugandhe vā'pi durgandhe mano ghrāṇeṣu jāyate /

tasmātpratyāharedetadātmanyava vaśaṃ nayet //4//

Whether there is a good or bad smell, the mind goes to it. Therefore, withdraw the mind from it (smell) and keep it under the control of the Self. -4.

मधुराम्लकतिक्तादिरसं गतं यदा मनः ।

तस्मात्प्रत्याहरेदेतदात्मन्येव वशं नयेत् ॥५॥

madhurāmlakatiktādirasaṃ gataṃ yadā manaḥ /

tasmātpratyāharedetadātmanyava vaśaṃ nayet //5//

Whenever the mind becomes attracted to sweet, sour, bitter and other (kinds) of tastes, withdraw it from them and bring it under the control of the Self. -5.

इति श्रीघेरण्डसंहितायां घेरण्डचण्डसंवादे

प्रत्याहारप्रयोगो नाम चतुर्थोपदेशः ॥

iti śrīgheraṇḍasamhitāyāṃ gheraṇḍacaṇḍasamvāde

pratyāhārāprayogo nāma caturthopadeśaḥ /

Thus ends the Fourth Chapter of *Gheraṇḍa Samhitā*

entitled *Pratyāhāra* Practice.

Chapter Five

Discourse On Prāṇāyāma

घेरण्ड उवाच ।

अथातः संप्रवक्ष्यामि प्राणायामस्य यद्विधिम् ।

यस्य साधनमात्रेण देवतुल्यो भवेन्नरः ॥१॥

gheraṇḍa uvāca /

athātaḥ sampravakṣyāmi prāṇāyāmasya yadviddhim /

yasya sādhanamātreṇa devatulyo bhvennaraḥ //1//

Sage *Gheraṇḍa* said: - Now I shall explain you about the rules of *prāṇāyāma*. By its mere practice, a man becomes similar to a god. -1.

आदौ स्थानं तथा कालं मिताहारं तथापरम् ।

नाडीशुद्धिं च ततः पश्चात्प्राणायामं च साधयेत् ॥२॥

ādau sthānaṃ tathā kālaṃ mitāhāraṃ tatha param /

nāḍīśuddhiṃ ca tataḥ paścātprāṇāyāmaṃ ca sādhayet //2//

First one should find a place and suitable time (for practice), eat in moderation and purify the *nāḍīs*. After that, he should practice *prāṇāyāma*. -2.

Place of Practice

दूरदेशे तथाऽरण्ये राजधान्यां जनान्तिके ।

योगारम्भं न कुर्वीत कृतश्चेत्सिद्धिहा भवेत् ॥३॥

dūradeśe tathā'raṇye rājadhānyāṃ janāntike /

yogārambhaṃ na kurvīta kṛtaścetsiddhihā bhavet //3//

One should not commence yogic practices in a far away land, in a forest, in a capital city or in the crowd. If one does so, he will not achieve *siddhi* (perfection). -3.

अविश्वासं दूरदेशे अरण्ये रक्षिवर्जितम् ।

लोकारण्ये प्रकाशश्च तस्मात् त्रीणि विवर्जयेत् ॥४॥

aviśvāsaṃ dūradeśe araṇye rakṣivarjitam /

lokāraṇye prakāśaśca tasmāt trīṇi vivarjayet //4//

One cannot believe people in a far away land. One is without protection in a forest. In the middle of dense population, one is open to public. Therefore, these three places should be avoided. -4.

सुदेशे धार्मिके राज्ये सुभिक्षे निरुपद्रवे ।

तत्रैकं कुटिरं कृत्वा प्राचीरैः परिवेष्टितम् ॥५॥

sudeśe dhārmike rājye subhikṣe nirupadrave /

kṛtvā tatraikaṃ kuṭīraṃ prācīraiḥ pariveṣṭitam //5//

In a good religious country where foods are sufficiently available in alms and is free from any disturbances, one should make a hut there and erect a wall around it. -5.

वापीकूपतडागं च प्राचीरमध्यवर्ति च ।

नात्युच्चं नातिनिम्नं च कुटिरं कीटवर्जितम् ॥६॥

vāpīkūpataḍāgaṃ ca prācīramadhyavarti ca /

nātyuccaṃ nātinimnaṃ ca kuṭīraṃ kīṭavarjitam //6//

There should be a well, a pond or a water source in the center of the boundary. The hut should be neither too high nor too low and be free from insects. -6.

सम्यग्गोमयलिप्तं च कुटिरं तत्र निर्मितम् ।

एवं स्थानेषु गुप्तेषु च प्राणायामं समभ्यसेत् ॥७॥

samyaggomayaliptaṃ ca kuṭīrantatra nirmitam /

evaṃ sthāneṣu gupteṣu prāṇāyāmaṃ samabhyaset //7//

The hut should be smeared well with cow-dung. In a hut built in this way located in a hidden place, one should practice *prāṇāyāma*. -7.

Time of Practice

हेमन्ते शिशिरे ग्रीष्मे वर्षायां च ऋतौ तथा ।

योगारम्भं न कुर्वीत कृते योगो हि रोगदः ॥८॥

hemante śiśire grīṣme varṣāyāṃ ca ṛtau tathā /

yogārambhaṃ na kurvīta kṛte yogo hi rogadaḥ //8//

One should not commence yogic practices during *hemanta* (winter), *śiśira* (cold), *grīṣma* (hot) and *varṣā* (rainy)seasons. If one does so in these seasons, the yoga indeed causes diseases for him. -8.

वसन्ते शरदि प्रोक्तं योगारम्भं समाचरेत् ।

तथा योगी भवेत् सिद्धो रोगान्मुक्तो भवेद् ध्रुवम् ॥९॥

vasante śaradi proktaṃ yogārambhaṃ samācaret /

tatha yogī bhavet siddho rogānmukto bhaved dhruvam //9//

It is said that one should begin the practice of yoga in spring (*vasanta*) and autumn (*śarada*) seasons. Thus, the yogi certainly becomes successful and free from diseases. -9.

चैत्रादिफाल्गुनान्ते च माघादिफाल्गुनान्तिके ।

द्वौ द्वौ मासौ ऋतुभागौ अनुभावश्चतुश्चतुः ॥१०॥

caitrādiphālgunānte ca māghādiphālgunāntike /

dvau dvau māsau ṛtubhāgau anubāvaścatuścatuḥ //10//

There are twelve months in a year from *caitrā* (March) to *phālguna* (February) and each season having two months duration follows in order starting from *māgha* to *phālguna*. But each season is also experienced for four months. -10.

वसन्तश्चैत्र वैशाखौ ज्येष्ठाषाढौ च ग्रीष्मकौ ।

वर्षा श्रावणभाद्राभ्यां शरदाश्विनकार्तिकौ ।

मार्गपौषौ च हेमन्तः शिशिरो माघफाल्गुनौ ॥११॥

vasantaścaitra vaiśākhau jyeṣṭhāṣāḍhā ca grīṣmakau /

varṣā śrāvaṇabhādrābhyāṃ śaradāśvinakārtikau /

mārgapauṣau ca hemantaḥ śiśiro māghaphālgunau //11//

Caitra and *vaiśākha* (March and April) is *vasanta* (spring); *jyeṣṭha āṣāḍha* (May and June) is *grīṣma* (summer); *śravaṇa* and *bhādrā* (July and August) is *varṣā* (rainy season); *āśvina* and *kārtika* (September and October) is *śarada* (autumn); *mārgaśīrṣa* and *pauṣa* (November and December) is *hemanta* (winter); and *māgha* to *phālguna* (January and February) is *śiśira* (cold). -11.

अनुभावं प्रवक्ष्यामि ऋतूनां च यथोदितम् ।

माघादिमाधवान्तेषु वसन्तानुभवं विदुः ॥१२॥

चैत्रादि चाषाढान्तं च निदाघानुभवं विदुः ।

आषाढादि चाश्विनान्तं प्रावृषानुभवं विदुः ॥१३॥

भाद्रादि मार्गशीर्षान्तं शरदोऽनुभवं विदुः ।

कार्तिकादिमाघमासान्तं हेमन्तानुभवं विदुः ।

मार्गादि चतुरो मासान् शिशिरानुभवं विदुः ॥१४॥

anubhāvam pravakṣyāmi ṛtūnām ca yothoditam /

māghādimādhavānteṣu vasantānubhavam viduḥ //12//

caitrādi cāṣāḍhāntam ca nidāghānubhavam viduḥ /

āṣāḍhādi cāśvināntam prāvṛṣānubhavam viduḥ //13//

bhādrādi mārgaśīrṣantam śarado'nubhavam viduḥ /

kārtikādimāghamāsāntam hemantānubhavam viduḥ /

mārgādi caturo māsān śiśirānubhavam vidūḥ //14//

Now I explain you about the seasons which are experienced as below. From *māgha* to *mādhava/vaiśākha* (January to April) spring is experienced; from *caitrā* to *āṣāḍha* (March to June) summer is experienced; from *āṣāḍha* to *āśvina* (June to September) monsoon is experienced; from *bhādra* to *mārgaśīrṣa* (August to November) autumn is experienced; from *kārtika* to *māgha* (October to January) winter is experienced; and from *mārgaśīrṣa* to *phālguna* (November to February) cold is experienced. -12-14.

वसन्ते वापि शरदि योगारम्भं समाचरेत् ।

तदा योगी भवेत्सिद्धो विनाऽऽयासेन कथ्यते ॥१५॥

vasante vāpi śaradi yogārambham samācaret /

tadā yogo bhavetsiddho vinā''yāsena kathyate //15//

It is said that yogic practices should be commenced either in *vasanta* (spring) or *śarada* (autumn). Thus, one attains success in his yogic practices without trouble. -15.

Moderation in Diet

मिताहारं विना यस्तु योगारम्भं तु कारयेत् ।

नानारोगो भवेत्तस्य किञ्चिद्योगो न सिध्यति ॥१६॥

mitāhāraṃ vinā yastu yogārambhaṃ tu kārayet /

nānārogo bhavettasya kiñcityogo na sidhyati //16//

One who does yogic practices without moderation in diet gets various diseases and certainly does not attain perfection/success in yoga. -16.

शाल्यन्नं यवपिष्टं वा गोधूमपिष्टकं तथा ।

मुद्गं माषचणकादि शुभ्रं च तुषवर्जितम् ॥१७॥

śālyannaṃ yavapiṣṭaṃ vā godhūmapiṣṭakaṃ tathā /

mudgaṃ māṣacaṇakādi śubhraṃ ca tuṣavarjitam //17//

One who practices yoga should eat food made from rice, barley or wheat flour and pulses like *mudga* (green beans), *māṣa* (black gram), *caṇaka* (chick peas), etc. which are clean and without husks. -17.

पटोलं पनसं मानं कक्कोलं च शुकाशाकम् ।

द्राढिकां कर्कटीं रम्भां डुम्बरीं कण्टकण्टकम् ॥१८॥

आमरम्भां बालरम्भां रम्भादण्डं च मूलकम् ।

वार्ताकीं मूलकम् ऋद्धिं योगी भक्षणमाचरेत् ॥१९॥

paṭolaṃ panasaṃ mānaṃ kakkolaṃ ca śukāśakam /

drāḍhikāṃ karkaṭīṃ rambhāṃ ḍumbarīṃ kaṇṭakaṇṭakam //18//

āmarambhāṃ bālarambhāṃ rambhādaṇḍaṃ ca mūlakam /

vārtākīṃ mūlakam ṛddhiṃ yogī bhakṣaṇamācaret //19//

A yogi can eat pointed gourd (trichosanthes dioica), jackfruit, root vegetables, berries, bitter gourd, cucumber, figs, plantain, plantain stem and roots, eggplants, radish and medicinal roots and fruits. -18-19.

बालशाकं कालशाकं तथा पटोलपत्रकम् ।

पञ्चशाकं प्रशंसीयाद्वास्तूकं हिलमोचिकाम् ॥२०॥

bālaśākam kālaśākam tathā poṭalapatrakam /

pañcaśākam praśamsīyādvāstūkam himalocikām //20//

Five green vegetables *bālaśāka, kālaśāka, poṭalapatra, vāstūka* and *himalocika* are recommended for a yogi. -20.

शुद्धं सुमधुरं स्निग्धमुदरार्धविवर्जितम् ।

भुज्यते सुरसं प्रीत्या मिताहारमिमं विदुः ॥२१॥

śuddham sumadhuram snigdham udarārdhavivarjitam /

bhujyate surasamprītyā mitāhāramimam viduḥ //21//

Eating pure, sweet and cool foods (cooked with ghee or butter); drinking good juices with pleasure and keeping half of the stomach empty is called moderation in diet by the wise. -21.

अन्नेन पूरयेदर्धं तोयेन तु तृतीयकम् ।

उदरस्य तुरीयांशं संरक्षेद्वायुचारणे ॥२२॥

annena pūrayedardham toyena tu tṛtīyakam /

udarasya turīyāmśam samrakṣedvāyucāraṇe //22//

Half of the stomach should be filled with food; the third quarter (of it) with water and *turīyāmśa* (the last part or fourth quarter) should be reserved for *vāyucāraṇa* (the movement of air). -22.

Forbidden Foods

कट्वम्लं लवणं तिक्तं भृष्टं च दधि तक्रकम् ।

शाकोत्कटं तथा मद्यं तालं च पनसं तथा ॥२३॥

kaṭvamlam lavaṇam tiktam bhṛṣṭam ca dadhi takrakam /

śākotkaṭaṃ tathā madyaṃ tālaṃ ca panasaṃ tathā //23//

While doing yogic practice for the first time, one should give up bitter, sour, salty, astringent and roasted food items, curd, buttermilk, heavy vegetables, wine, palm nuts and over-ripe jack fruits. -23.

कुलत्थं मसूरं पाण्डुं कूष्माण्डं शाकदण्डकम् ।

तुम्बीकोलकपित्थं च कण्टबिल्वं पलाशकम् ॥२४॥

kulatthaṃ masuraṃ pāṇḍuṃ kūṣmāṇḍaṃ śākadaṇḍakam /

tumbīkolakapitthaṃ ca kaṇṭabilbaṃ palāśakam //24//

One should avoid horse gram, lentils, *pāṇḍu* (a kind of fruit), pumpkin, vegetable stems, gourds, *kaṇṭabilba* (feronia elephantum) and *palāśaka* (butea frondosa). -24.

कदम्बं जम्बीरं बिम्बं लकुचं लशुनं विषम् ।

कामरङ्गं पियालं च हिङ्गुशाल्मलिकेमुकम् ॥२५॥

kadambaṃ jambīraṃ bimbaṃ lakucaṃ laśunaṃ viṣam /

kāmaraṅgaṃ piyālaṃ ca hiṅguśālmalīkemukam //25//

Also he should avoid fruit like berries, limes, garlic and onions, asafoetida, *śālmalī* and *kemuka*. -25.

योगारम्भे वर्जयेच्च पथस्त्रीवह्निसेवनम् ।

नवनीतं घृतं क्षीरं गुडं शर्करादि चैक्षवम् ॥२६॥

पक्करम्भां नारिकेलं दाडिम्बमशिवासवम् ।

द्राक्षां तु लवनीं धात्रीं रसमम्लविवर्जितम् ॥२७॥

yogārambhe varjayecca pathastrivahnisevanam /

navanītaṃ ghṛtaṃ kṣīraṃ guḍaṃ śarkarādi caikṣavam //26//

pakvarambhāṃ nārikelaṃ dāḍimbamaśivāsavam /

drākṣāṃ tu lavalīṃ dhātriṃ rasamamlavivarjitam //27//

When one begins yogic practice for the first time, he should avoid travelling, the company of the women and serving the fire (for heating the body). He should also avoid fresh butter, clarified butter, milk, sugar-candy, jaggery, ripe banana, coconut, pomegranate, grapes, *lavalī* fruit, myrobalans and acidic juices. – 26-27.

एलाजातिलवङ्गं च पौरुषं जम्बु जाम्बलम् ।

हरीतकीं खर्जूरं च योगी भक्षणमाचरेत् ॥२८॥

लघुपाकं प्रियं स्निग्धं तथा धातुप्रपोषणम् ।

मनोऽभिलषितं योग्यं योगी भोजनमाचरेत् ॥२९॥

elājātilavaṅgaṃ ca pauruṣaṃ jambu jāmbalam /

harītakīṃ kharjūraṃ ca yogī bhakṣaṇamācaret //28//

laghupākaṃ priyaṃ snigdhaṃ tathā dhātuprapoṣaṇam /

mano 'bhilaṣitaṃ yogyaṃ yogī bhojanamācaret //29//

A yogi can eat cardamom, nutmeg, cloves, stimulants, *harītakī* and dates. He should eat easily digestible, agreeable and cool foods which nourish the humors of the body and appeal to his mind. -28-29.

काठिन्यं दुरितं पूतिमुष्णं पर्युषितं तथा ।

अतिशीतं चाति चोष्णं भक्ष्यं योगी विवर्जयेत् ॥३०॥

kāṭhinyaṃ duritaṃ pūtimuṣṇaṃ paryuṣitaṃ tathā /

atiśītaṃ cāti coṣṇaṃ bhakṣyaṃ yogī vivarjayet //30//

He should avoid the foods which are hard (difficult to digest), rotten, stale, heating, very cold and very hot. -30.

प्रातःस्नानोपवासादिकायक्लेशविधिं तथा ।

एकाहारं निराहारं यामान्ते च न कारयेत् ॥३१॥

prātaḥsnānopavāsādi kāyakleśavidhiṃ tathā /

ekāhāraṃ nirāhāraṃ yāmānte ca na kārayet //31//

He should not take early morning baths, do fasting or do any activity that causes pain for the body. He should avoid eating only once a day, not eating at all and eating at the end of every three hours (between meals). -31.

एवं विधिविधानेन प्राणायामं समाचरेत् ।

आरम्भे प्रथमे कुर्यात्क्षीराज्यं नित्यभोजनम् ।

मध्याह्ने चैव सायाह्ने भोजनद्वयमाचरेत् ॥३२॥

evaṃ vidhividhānena prāṇāyāmaṃ samācaret /

ārambhe prathame kuryātkṣīrājyaṃ nityabhojanam /

madhyāhne caiva sāyāhne bhokjanadvayamāacaret //32//

According to the rules as specified above, one should begin *prāṇāyāma* practice. Before beginning *prāṇāyāma* practice, he should take food with milk and ghee daily and eat two meals a day, one at noon and the next in the evening. -32.

Purification of Nāḍī

कुशासने मृगाजिने व्याघ्राजिने च कम्बले ।

स्थलासने समासीनः प्राङ्मुखो वाप्युदङ्मुखः ।

नाडीशुद्धिं समासाद्य प्राणायामं समभ्यसेत् ॥३३॥

kuśāsane mṛgājine vyāghrājine ca kambale /

sthalāsane samāsīnaḥ prāṅmukho vāpyudaṅmukhaḥ /

nāḍīśuddhiṃ samāsādhya prāṇāyāmaṃ samabhyaset //33//

One should sit on a seat of *kuśa* (a sacred grass) or deer skin or a tiger skin or a blanket facing east or north. Having purified the *nāḍīs* first, he should do the practice of *prāṇāyāma*. -33.

चण्डकापालिरुवाच ।

नाडीशुद्धिं कथं कुर्यान्नाडीशुद्धिस्तु कीदृशी ।

तत्सर्वं श्रोतुमिच्छामि तद्वदस्व दयानिधे ॥३४॥

caṇḍakapāliruvāca /

nāḍīśuddhiṃ kathaṃ kuryānnāḍīśuddhistu kīdṛśī /

tatsarvaṃ śrotumicchāmi tatvadasva dayānidhe //34//

Caṇḍakapāli asked: - How is purification of *nāḍīs* done? What is its form? I want to hear all about these. O ocean of kindness, please tell me about it. -34.

घेरण्ड उवाच ।

मलाकुलासु नाडीषु मारुतो नैव गच्छति ।

प्राणायामः कथं सिध्येत्तत्त्वज्ञानं कथं भवेत् ।

तस्मादादौ नडीशुद्धिं प्राणायामं ततोऽभ्यसेत् ॥३५॥

gheraṇḍa uvāca /

malākulāsu nāḍīṣu māruto naiva gacchati /

prāṇāyāmaḥ kathaṃ siddhayetatvajñānaṃ kathaṃ bhavet /

tasmādādau nāḍīśuddhiṃ prāṇāyāmaṃ tato 'bhyaset //35//

Sage *Gheraṇḍa* replied: - The air cannot go through the *nāḍīs* when they are full of impurities. In this condition, how can *prāṇāyāma* be perfected? How can *tatvajñāna* (the real knowledge) arise? Therefore, first of all one must purify the *nāḍīs*, and then he should practice *prāṇāyāma*. -35.

नाडीशुद्धिर्द्विधा प्रोक्ता समनुर्निर्मनुस्तथा ।

बीजेन समनुं कुर्यान्निर्मनुं धौतिकर्मणा ॥३६॥

nāḍīśuddhirdvidhā proktā samanurnirmanustathā /

bījena samanuṃ kuryānnirmanuṃ dhautikarmaṇā //36//

Purification of *nāḍīs* is of two types. They are *samanu* and *nirmanu*. *Samanu* is performed with *bīja mantra*. *Nirmanu* is performed with the practice of *dhauti karma*. -36.

धौतिकर्म पुरा प्रोक्तं षट्कर्मसाधने यथा ।

शृ ुणुष्व समनुं चण्ड नाडीशुद्धिर्यथा भवेत् ॥३७॥

dhautikarma purā proktaṃ ṣaṭkarmasādhane yathā /

śruṇuṣva samanuṃ caṇda nāḍīśuddhiryathā bhavet //37//

The *dhautikarma* has already been described in the practice of *ṣatkarma* sādhanā (the six yogic cleansing practices). O *Caṇda*, now listen to the *samanu* method through which the *nāḍīs* are purified. -37.

उपविश्यासने योगी पद्मासनं समाचरेत् ।

गुर्वादिन्यासनं कुर्याद्यथैव गुरुभाषितम् ।

नाडीशुद्धिं प्रकुर्वीत प्राणायामविशुद्धये ॥३८॥

upaviśyāsane yogī padmāsanaṃ samācaret /

gurvādinyāsanaṃ kuryād yathaiva gurubhāṣitam /

nāḍīśuddhiṃ prakurvīta prāṇāyāmaviśuddhaye //38//

After sitting on a seat, a yogi should assume *padmāsana* and perform *gurvādinyāsa* (invocation of the guru, etc., by rotating awareness on various parts of the body with specific *mantras*). Then according to the instructions of the guru, practice purification of the *nāḍīs* for attaining perfection in *prāṇāyāma*. -38.

वायुबीजं ततो ध्यात्वा धूम्रवर्णं सतेजसम् ।

चन्द्रेण पूरयेद्वायुं बीजषोडशकैः सुधीः ॥३९॥

चतुःषष्ट्या मात्रया च कुम्भकेनैव धारयेत् ।

द्वात्रिंशन्मात्रया वायुं सूर्यनाड्या च रेचयेत् ॥४०॥

vāyubījaṃ tato dhyātvā dhūmravarṇaṃ satejasam /

candreṇa pūrayedvāyuṃ vījaṃ ṣoḍaśakaiḥ śudhiḥ //39//

catuḥṣaṣṭyā mātrayā ca kumbhakenaiva dhārayet /

dvātrimśanmātrayā vāyuṃ sūryanāḍyā ca recayet //40//

Meditating on *vāyubīja mantra* '*yaṃ*' with its bright smoke color, perform *pūraka* (inhalation) through the *candra nāḍī* (left nostril) repeating the *bīja mantra* sixteen times. Thus, after inhalation perform *kumbhaka* (retention of breath) repeating the *mantra* sixty-four times. then perform *rechaka* (exhalation) through *sūryanāḍī* (right nostril) repeating the *mantra* thirty-two times. -39-40.

नाभिमूलाद्वह्निमुत्थाप्य ध्यायेत्तेजोऽवनीयुतम् ।

वह्निबीजषोडशेन सूर्यनाड्या च पूरयेत् ॥४१॥

चतुःषष्ट्या मात्रया च कुम्भकेनैव धारयेत् ।

द्वात्रिंशन्मात्रया वायुं शशिनाड्या च रेचयेत् ॥४२॥

nābhimūlādvahnimutthāpya dhyāyettejo'vanīyutam /

vahnibījaṣoḍaśena sūryanāaḍyā ca pūrayet //41//

catuḥṣaṣṭyā mātrayā ca kumbhakenaiva dhārayet /

dvātriśanmātrayā vāyuṃ śaśināḍyā ca recayet //42//

Raising the fire element from the navel center, concentrate on its light associated with the earth element. Repeating the *raṃ bīja* of fire element sixteen times, inhale through *sūryanāḍī* (right nostril), hold the breath through *kumbhaka* repeating it sixty-four times and then exhale through the *śaśi nāḍī* (left nostril) repeating the *mantra* thirty-two times. -41-42.

नासाग्रे शशधृग्बिम्बं ध्यात्वा ज्योत्स्नासमन्वितम् ।

ठं बीजं षोडशेनैव इडया पूरयेन्मरुत् ॥४३॥

चतुःषष्ट्या मात्रया च वं बीजेनैव धारयेत् ।

अमृतं प्लावितं ध्यात्वा नाडीधौतिं विभावयेत् ।

लकारेण द्वात्रिंशेन दृढं भाव्यं विरेचयेत् ॥४४॥

nāsāgre śaśadhṛgbimbaṃ dhyātvā jyotsnāsamanvitam /

ṭhaṃ bījaṃ ṣoḍaśenaiva iḍayā pūrayenmarut //43//

catuḥṣaṣṭyā mātrayā ca vaṃ bījenaiva dhārayet /

amṛtaṃ plāvitaṃ dhyātvā nāḍīdhautiṃ vibhāvayet /

lakāreṇa dvātrimśena dṛḍhaṃ bhāvyaṃ virecayet //44//

Concentrating on the image of the moon with its luminous reflection on the tip of the nose, inhale through the left nostril repeating the *bīja mantra* 'ṭhaṃ' sixteen times. Hold the breath by *kumbhaka* repeating the *bīja mantra* 'vaṃ' sixty-four times. Perceive the flow of nectar from the moon at the tip of the nose and purify all the *nāḍīs*. Then exhale through the right nostril by repeating the *bīja mantra* 'laṃ' thirty-two times. -43-44.

एवंविधां नाडीशुद्धिं कृत्वा नाडीं विशोधयेत् ।

दृढो भूत्वाऽऽसनं कृत्वा प्राणायामं समाचरेत् ॥४५॥

evamvidhāṃ nāḍīśuddhiṃ kṛtvā nāḍīṃ viśodhayet /

dhṛḍhobhūtvā"sanaṃ kṛtvā prāṇāyāmaṃ samācaret //45//

Purify the *nāḍīs* through these specified methods. After purifying the *nāḍīs*, be firmly seated in an *āsana* and begin the practice of *prāṇāyāma*. -45.

Types of Kumbhaka

सहितः सूर्यभेदश्च उज्जायी शीतली तथा ।

भस्त्रिका भ्रामरी मूर्च्छा केवली चाष्टकुम्भकाः ॥४६॥

sahitaḥ sūryabhedaśca ujjāyī śītalī tathā /

bhastrikā bhrāmarī mūrcchā kevalī cāṣṭakumbhakā //46//

There are eight types of *praṇāyāmas*. They are *sahita, sūrya bheda, ujjāyī, śītalī, bhastrikā, bhrāmarī, mūrcchā* and *kevalī.* -46.

Sahita Prāṇāyāma

सहितो द्विविधः प्रोक्तः सगर्भश्च निगर्भकः ।

सगर्भो बीजमुच्चार्य निगर्भो बीज वर्जितः ॥४७॥

sahita dvividhaḥ proktaḥ sagarbhśca nigarbhakaḥ /

sagarbho bījamuccārya nigarbho bīja varjitaḥ //47//

*Sahita prāṇāyāma*is of two types: *sagarbha* and *nigarbha. Bīja mantra* is repeated in *sagarbhaprāṇāyāma. Nigarbhaprāṇāyāma* is done without *bīja mantra.* -47.

Sagarbha Prāṇāyāma

प्राणायामं सगर्भं च प्रथमं कथयामि ते ।

सुखासने चोपविश्य प्राङ्मुखो वाऽप्युदङ्मुखः ।

ध्यायेद् विधिं रजोगुणं रक्तवर्णमवर्णकम् ॥४८॥

prāṇāyāmaṃ sagarbhaṃ ca prathamaṃ kathayāmi te /

sukhāsane copāviśya praṅmukho vā'pyudaṅmukhaḥ /

dhyāyed vidhiṃ rajoguṇaṃ raktavarṇamavarṇam //48//

First of all, I shall tell you about *sagarbha prāṇāyāma.* Sit in *sukhāsana* (easy pose) facing east or north and meditate on red colored *Brahmā,* full of *rajas guṇa* with the letter '*a*' as its *bīja mantra.* -48.

इडया पूरयेद्वायुं मात्रया षोडशैः सुधीः ।

पूरकान्ते कुम्भकाद्ये कर्तव्यस्तूड्डियानकः ॥४९॥

सत्त्वमयं हरिं ध्यात्वा उकारं कृष्णवर्णकम् ।

चतुःषष्ट्या च मात्रया कुम्भकेनैव धारयेत् ॥५०॥

तमोमयं शिवं ध्यात्वा मकारं शुक्लवर्णकम् ।

द्वात्रिंशन्मात्रया चैव रेचयेद्विधिना पुनः ॥५१॥

iḍayā pūrayedvāyuṃ mātrayā ṣoḍaśaiḥ sudhiḥ /

pūrakānte kumbhakādye kartavyastūḍḍiyānakaḥ //49//

satvamayaṃ hariṃ dhyātvā ukāraṃ kṛṣṇavarṇakam /

catuḥṣaṣṭyā ca mātrayā kumbhakenaiva dhārayet //50//

tamomayaṃ śivaṃ dhyātvā makāraṃ śuklavarṇakam /

dvātrimśanmātrayā caiva recayedvidhinā punaḥ //51//

Inhale through the left nostril repeating *bīja mantra* 'a' sixteen times. At the end of inhalation and before *kumbhaka*, perform *uḍḍiyāna bandha*. Then hold the breath repeating *bīja mantra* 'u' sixty-four times and meditate on dark colored *Hari* full of *satvaguṇa*. Then again exhale repeating the *bīja mantra* 'm' thirty-two times meditating on bright colored *Śiva* full of *tamas guṇa*. -49-51.

पुनः पिङ्गलयाऽऽपूर्य कुम्भकेनैव धारयेत् ।

इडया रेचयेत्पश्चात्तद्बीजेन क्रमेण तु ॥५२॥

अनुलोमविलोमेन वारं वारं च साधयेत् ।

पूरकान्ते कुम्भकान्तं धृतनासापुटद्वयम् ।

कनिष्ठाकानामिकाङ्गुष्ठैः तर्जनी मध्यमे विना ॥५३॥

punaḥ piṅgalayā"pūrya kumbhakenaiva dhārayet /

iḍayā recayetpaścāt tadbījena krameṇa tu //52//

anulomavilomena vāram vāraṃ ca sādhayet /

pūrakānte kumbhakāntaṃ dhṛtanāsāpuṭadvayam /

kaniṣṭhākānāmikāṅguṣṭhaiḥ tarjani madhyame vinā //53//

Again inhale through the right nostril, retain the breath and exhale through the left nostril repeating the *bīja mantras* in the same way/order as mentioned before. In this way, practice *anuloma viloma* (alternate nostril breathing) again and again. After the end of inhalation till the end of *kumbhaka*, close both nostrils, the right (nostril) with the thumb and the left (nostril) with the ring finger and little finger without (using) the index and middle fingers. -52-53.

Nigarbha Prāṇāyāma

प्राणायामो निगर्भस्तु विना बीजेन जायते ।

वामजानूपरिन्यस्तं वामपाणितलं भ्रमेत् ।

एकादिशतपर्यन्तं पूरकुम्भकरेचनम् ॥५४॥

prāṇāyāmo nigarbhastu vinā bījena jāyate /

vāmajānūparinyastaṃ vāmapāṇitalaṃ bhramet /

ekādiśataparyantaṃ pūrakumbhakarecanam //54//

Practice of *nigarbha prāṇāyāma* is done without *bīja mantras*. The left hand is moved around on the left knee (for the count) of *prāṇāyāma* during *pūraka, kumbhaka* and *recaka* (inhalation, retention and exhalation) from one to hundred. -54.

उत्तमा विंशतिर्मात्रा षोडशी मात्रा मध्यमा ।

अधमा द्वादशी मात्रा प्राणायामास्त्रिधा स्मृताः ॥५५॥

uttamā viṃśatirmātrā ṣoḍaśī mātrā madhyamā /

adhamā dvādaśi mātrā prāṇāyāmāstridhā smṛtā //55//

The highest *prāṇāyāma* has twenty *mātrās* (i.e. the ratio of counts is 20:80:40), the medium has sixteen *mātrās* (i.e. the ratio of counts is 16:64:32) and the lowest has twelve *mātrās* (i.e. the ratio of counts is 12:48:24). Thus, *prāṇāyāma* is considered of three types. -55.

अधमाज्जायते घर्मो मेरुकम्पश्च मध्यमात् ।

उत्तमाच्च भूमित्यागस्त्रिविधं सिद्धिलक्षणम् ॥५६॥

adhamājjāyate gharmo merukampaśca madhyamāt /

uttamācca bhūmityāgastrividhaṃ siddhilakṣaṇam //56//

The lowest type of *prāṇāyāma* produces heat or perspiration in the body. The medium type of *prāṇāyāma* causes trembling of the spinal column. By the highest type of *prāṇāyāma*, one gives up the ground (levitates). These three results (of *prāṇāyāma* practice) are considered as signs of perfection. -56.

प्राणायामात् खेचरत्वं प्राणायामात् रोगनाशनम् ।

प्राणायामात् बोधयेच्छक्तिं प्राणायामात् मनोन्मनी ।

आनन्दो जायते चित्ते प्राणायामी सुखी भवेत् ॥५७॥

prāṇāyāmāt khecaratvaṃ prāṇāyāmāt roganaśanam /

prāṇāyāmāt bodhayecchaktiṃ prāṇāyāmāt manonmanī /

ānando jāyate citte prāṇāyāmī sukhī bhavet //57//

Through the practice of *prāṇāyāma*, travelling ability in space is attained. Diseases are destroyed by the *prāṇāyāmā*. *Kuṇḍalinī śakti* is awakened through the practice of *prāṇāyāma*. *Manonmanī* (a blissful state of mind) is achieved by the *prāṇāyāma*. Through *prāṇāyāma* practice, mind becomes *ānanda* (joyful). One who practices *prāṇāyāma* becomes happy. -57.

Sūryabheda Prāṇāyāma

कथितं सहितं कुम्भं सूर्यभेदनकं शृणु ।

पूरयेत्सूर्यनाड्या च यथाशक्ति बहिर्मरुत् ॥५८॥

धारयेद्बहुयत्नेन कुम्भकेन जलन्धरैः ।

यावत्स्वेदं नखकेशाभ्यां तावत्कुर्वन्तु कुम्भकम् ॥५९॥

kathitaṃ sahitaṃ kumbhaṃ sūryabhedanakaṃ śṛṇu /

pūrayet sūryanāḍyā ca yathāśaktiṃ bahirmarut //58//

dhārayedbahuyatnena kumbhakena jalandharaiḥ /

yāvatsvedaṃ nakhakeśābhyāṃ tāvatkurvantu kumbhakam //59//

Sahita kumbhaka has already been explained. Now pay attention to *sūryabheda*. Inhale deeply as far as possible through the right nostril and hold the breath with all the effort performing *jālandhara bandha* until the body perspires from the nails to the hairs on the head. -58-59.

Prāṇa Vāyus

प्राणोऽपानः समानश्चोदानव्यानौ तथैव च ।

नागः कूर्मश्च कृकरो देवदत्तो धनञ्जयः ॥६०॥

prāṇo'pānaḥ samānaścodānavyānau tathaiva ca /

nāgaḥ kūrmaśca kṛkaro devadatto dhanañjayaḥ //60//

There are ten *prāṇa vāyus*. They are *prāṇa, apāna, samāna, udāna, vyāna, nāga, kūrma, kṛkara, devadatta* and *dhanañjaya*. -60.

Locations of Prāṇa Vāyus

हृदि प्राणो वहेन्नित्यमपानो गुदमण्डले ।

समानो नाभिदेशे तु उदानः कण्ठमध्यगः ॥६१॥

व्यानो व्याप्य शरीरे तु प्रधानाः पञ्च वायवः ।

प्राणाद्याः पञ्च विख्याता नागाद्याः पञ्च वायवः ॥६२॥

hṛdi prāṇo vahennityamapāno gudamaṇḍale /

samāno nābhideśe tu udānaḥ kaṇṭhamadhyagaḥ //61//

vyāno vyāpya śarīre tu pradhānāḥ pañca vāyavaḥ /

prāṇādyāḥ pañca vikhyātā nāgādyāḥ pañca vāyavaḥ //62//

Prāṇa always flows in the heart, *apāna* in the region of the anus, *samāna* in the navel region, *udāna* in the middle of the throat and *vyāna* is pervasive in the whole body. These five are known as the main *prāṇas. Nāga*, etc., are the five sub-*prāṇa vayus.* -62.

तेषामपि च पञ्चानां स्थानानि च वदाम्यहम् ।

उद्गारे नाग आख्यातः कूर्मस्तून्मीलने स्मृतः ॥६३॥

कृकरः क्षुत्कृते ज्ञेयो देवदत्तो विजृम्भणे ।

न जहाति मृते क्वापि सर्वव्यापी धनञ्जयः ॥६४॥

teṣāmapi ca pañcānāṃ sthānāni ca vadāmyaham /

udgāre nāga ākhyātaḥ kūrmastūnmīlane smṛtaḥ //63//

kṛkaraḥ kṣutkṛte jñeyo devadatto vijṛmbhaṇe /

na jahāti mṛte kvāpi sarvavyāpī dhanañjayaḥ //64//

Now I tell you the places of these five sub-*prāṇa vayus*. It is considered that *Nāga* presents in belching, *kūrma* in opening the eyes, *kṛkara* in sneezing; *devadatta* in yawning and *dhanañjaya*, all pervasive one, does not leave the body even after death. -63-64.

नागो गृह्णाति चैतन्यं कूर्मश्चैव निमेषणम् ।

क्षुत्तृषं कृकरश्चैव जृम्भणं चतुर्थेन तु ।

भवेद्धनञ्जयाच्छब्दं क्षणमात्रं न निःसरेत् ॥६५॥

nāgo gṛhṇāti caitanyaṃ kūrmaścaiva nimeṣaṇam /

kṣuttṛṣaṃ kṛkaraścaiva jṛmbhaṇaṃ caturthena tu /

bhaveddhanañjayācchabdaṃ kṣaṇamātraṃ na niḥsaret //65//

From *nāga* consciousness, from *kūrma* blinking (of the eyes), from *kṛkara* hunger and thirst and from *devadatta* yawning are produced. Sound is produced through *dhanañjaya* which does not leave the body even for a moment. -65.

सर्वे ते सूर्यसम्भिन्ना नाभिमूलात्समुद्धरेत् ।

इडया रेचयेत्पश्चाद्धैर्येणाखण्डवेगतः ॥६६॥

पुनः सूर्येण चाकृष्य कुम्भयित्वा यथाविधि ।

रेचयित्वा साधयेत्तु क्रमेण च पुनः पुनः ॥६७॥

sarve te sūryasambhinnā nābhimūlāt samuddharet /

iḍaya recayet paścād dhairyeṇākhaṇḍavegataḥ //66//

punaḥ sūryeṇa cākṛsya kumbhayitvā yathāvidhi /

recayitvā sādhayettu krameṇa ca punaḥ punaḥ //67//

Seperating these *prāṇa vayus* with the help of *sūryanāḍī* during practice, raise *samāna vāyu* which comes from the root of the navel. Then exhale slowly and continuously through the left nostril with patience. Again inhale through the right nostril, hold the breath as per the specified method, and exhale through left nostil. Repeat this process of practice again and again. -66-67.

कुम्भकः सूर्यभेदस्तु जरामृत्युविनाशकः ।

बोधयेत्कुण्डलीं शक्तिं देहानलविवर्धनम् ।

इति ते कथितं चण्ड सूर्यभेदनमुत्तमम् ॥६८॥

kumbhakaḥ sūryabhedastu jarāmṛtyuvināśakaḥ /

bodhayetkuṇḍalīṃ śaktiṃ dehānalavivardhanam /

iti te kathitaṃ caṇḍa sūryabhedanamuttamam //68//

This is *sūryabheda kumbhaka*, the destroyer of old age and death. It awakens the *kuṇḍalinī śakti* and increases the fire in the body. O Caṇḍa! I have told/taught you the excellent *prāṇāyāma* called *sūrya bheda*. -68.

Ujjāyī Prāṇāyāma

नासाभ्यां वायुमाकृष्य मुखमध्ये च धारयेत् ।

हृद्गलाभ्यां समाकृष्य वायुं वक्त्रे च धारयेत् ॥६९॥

मुखं प्राक्षल्य सम्वन्द्य कुर्याज्जालन्धरं ततः ।

आशक्ति कुम्भकं कृत्वा धारयेदविरोधतः ॥७०॥

nāsābhyāṃ vāyumākṛsya mukhamadhye ca dhārayet /

hṛdgalābhyāṃ samākṛsya vāyuṃ vaktre ca dhārayet //69//

mukhaṃ prakṣālya samvandya kuryājjālandharaṃ tataḥ /

āśakti kumbhakam kṛtvā dhārayedavirodhataḥ //70//

Inhaling the air through both nostrils, pull the internal air from the heart and throat and hold it in the mouth. After washing the mouth (with the air), perform *jālandhara bandha*. Hold the breath with *kumbhaka* according to capacity without causing any hindrance. -69-70.

उज्जायी कुम्भकं कृत्वा सर्वकार्याणि साधयेत् ।

न भवेत्कफरोगश्च क्रूरवायुरजीर्णकम् ॥७१॥

आमवातः क्षयः कासो ज्वरः प्लीहा न विद्यते ।

जरामृत्युविनाशाय चोज्जायीं साधयेन्नरः ॥७२॥

ujjāyī kumbhakam kṛtvā sarvakāryaṇī sādhayet /

na bhavet kapharogaśca krūravāyurajīrṇakam //71//

āmavātaḥ kṣayaḥ kāso jvaraḥ plīhā na vidyate /

jarāmṛtyuvināśāya cojjāyīṃ sādhayennaraḥ //72//

All works are accomplished by the practice of *ujjāyī kumbhaka*. *Kapha* (phlegm), *krūra vāyu* (air or nervous related disorders) and digestive disorders do not occur. Dysentery, tuberculosis, cough, fever and spleen disorders do not exist. A person should perfect *ujjāyī kumbhaka* in order to destroy old age and death. -71-72.

Śītalī Prāṇāyāma

जिह्वया वायुमावृष्य उदरे पूरयेच्छनै. ।

क्षणं च कुम्भकं कृत्वा नासाभ्यां रेचयेत्पुनः ॥७३॥

jihvayā vāyumākṛṣya udare purayecchanaiḥ /

kṣaṇaṃ ca kumbhakaṃ kṛtvā nāsābhyāṃ recayet punaḥ //73//

Pulling in the air through the tongue (rounded), slowly fill up the abdomen. Holding the breath for a short time, exhale it through both nostrils. -73.

सर्वदा साधयेद्योगी शीतलीकुम्भकं शुभम् ।

अजीर्णं कफपित्तं च नैव तस्य प्रजायते ॥७४॥

sarvadā sādhayedyogī śītalīkumbhakaṃ śubham /

ajīrṇaṃ kaphapittaṃ ca naiva tasya prajāyate //74//

A yogi should always practice this auspicious *śītalī kumbhaka*. By doing this practice, digestive disorders and *kapha* (phlegm) and *pitta* (bile) disorders do not appear. -74.

Bhastrikā Prāṇāyāma

भस्त्रैव लोहकाराणां यथाक्रमेण सम्भ्रमेत् ।

तथा वायुं च नासाभ्यामुभाभ्यां चालयेच्छनैः ॥७५॥

bhastraiva lauhakārāṇāṃ yathākrameṇa sambhramet /

tathā vāyuṃ ca nāsābhyāmubhābhyāṃ cālayecchanaiḥ //75//

Just like the (expanding and contracting) movements of the bellows of a blacksmith, inhale slowly and then exhale slowly through both nostrils. -75.

एवं विंशतिवारं च कृत्वा कुर्याच्च कुम्भकम् ।

तदन्ते चालयेद्वायुं पूर्वोक्तं च यथाविधि ॥७६॥

त्रिवारं साधयेदेनं भस्त्रिकाकुम्भकं सुधीः ।

न च रोगो न च क्लेश आरोग्यं च दिने दिने ॥७७॥

evam vimśativāraṃ ca kṛtvā kuryācca kumbhakam /

tadante calayedvāyuṃ pūrvoktaṃ ca yathāvidhi //76//

trivāraṃ sādhayedenaṃ bhastrikākumbhakaṃ śudhīḥ //

na ca rogo na ca kleśa arogyaṃ ca dine dine //77//

After repeating it twenty times, hold the breath and then practice this breath movement as per the prescribed method explained above. A wise yogi should practice this *bhastrikā kumbhaka* three rounds. Through its practice, diseases and afflictions do not appear and good health is attained everyday. -76-77.

Bhrāmarī Prāṇāyāma

अर्धरात्रे गते योगी जन्तूनां शब्दवर्जिते ।

कर्णौ पिधाय हस्ताभ्यां कुर्यात्पूरककुम्भकम् ॥७८॥

ardharātre gate yogī jantūnāṃ śabdavarjite /

karṇau pidhāya hastābhyāṃ kuryātpūrakakumbhakam //78//

After midnight, in a place where there are not any sounds of living beings, a yogi should practice *pūraka* (inhalation) and *kumbhaka* (retention) closing the ears with the hands. -78.

श्रृणुयाद्दक्षिणे कर्णे नादमन्तर्गतं शुभम् ।

प्रथमं झिङ्झिनादं च वंशीनादं ततः परम् ॥७९॥

मेघझर्झरभ्रामरी घण्टाकास्यं ततः परम् ।

तुरीभेरीमृदङ्गादि निनादानेकदुन्दुभिः ॥८०॥

śṛṇuyāddakṣiṇe karṇe nādamantargataṃ śubham /

prathamaṃ jhiñjhinādaṃ ca vaṃśinādaṃ tataḥ param //79//

meghajharjharabhrāmarī ghaṇṭākāsyaṃ tataḥ param /

turībherīmṛdaṅgādi ninādānekadundubhiḥ //80//

He then hears auspicious internal sounds in his right ear. First the sound of a cricket (grasshopper), then the sound of a flute, then the thundering sound of clouds, then the sound of a drum, then of a bee, then of bell, then of big metal gongs, then of a trumpet, a kettle drum, a drum and other kinds of drums. -79-80.

एवं नानाविधो नादो जायते नित्यमभ्यसात् ।

अनाहतस्य शब्दस्य तस्य शब्दस्य यो ध्वनिः ॥८१॥

ध्वनेरन्तर्गतं ज्योतिर्ज्योतिरन्तर्गतं मनः ।

तन्मनो विलयं याति तद्विष्णोः परमं पदम् ।

एवं भ्रामरीसंसिद्धिः समाधिसिद्धिमाप्नुयात् ॥८२॥

evaṃ nānāvidho nādo jāyate nityamabhyāsāt /

anāhatasya śabdasya tasya śabdasya yo dhvaniḥ //81//

dhvanerantargataṃ jyotirjyotirantargataṃ manaḥ /

tanmano vilayaṃ yāti tadviṣṇoḥ paramaṃ padam /

evaṃ bhrāmarīsamsiddhiḥ samādhisiddhimāpnuyāt //82//

Thus, one hears various sounds through regular practice. The sound that comes from *anāhata* has its resonance. In that resonance there is a light. The mind should be absorbed in that light. When the mind is dissolved into it, one attains the supreme seat of *Viṣṇu*. So by duly perfecting *bhrāmarī kumbhaka*, one achieves *siddhi* (perfection) in *samādhi*. -81.82.

Mūrcchā Prāṇāyāma

सुखेन कुम्भकं कृत्वा मनश्च भ्रुवोरन्तरम् ।

सन्त्यज्य विषयान्सर्वान्मनोमूर्च्छा सुखप्रदा ।

आत्मनि मनसो योगादानन्दो जायते ध्रुवम् ॥८३॥

sukhena kumbhakaṃ kṛtvā manaśca bhruvorantaram /

santyajya viṣayānsarvānmanomūrcchā sukhapradā /

ātmani manaso yogādānando jāyate dhruvam //83//

Holding the breath with *kumbhaka* comfortably, withdraw the mind from all sense-objects and fix it in the middle of the eyebrows. This causes *manomūrcchā* (literally, a fainted or an absent state of the mind, a state similar to *Samādhi*) and bestows happiness. By the yoga of joining the mind with the *Ātman*, a blissful state is certainly attained. -83.

Kevalī Prāṇāyāma

हङ्कारेण बहिर्याति सःकारेण विशेत्पुनः ।

षड्शतानि दिवारात्रौ सहस्राण्येकविंशतिः ।

अजपां नाम गायत्रीं जीवो जपति सर्वदा ॥८४॥

haṅkāreṇa bahiryāti saḥkāreṇa viśetpunaḥ /

ṣaṭsatāni divārātrau sahasrāṇyekavimśatiḥ /

ajapāṃ nāma gāyatrīṃ jīvo japati sarvadā //84//

A *jīva* (living being) exhales with *ham* sound and inhales with *sa* sound in every breath. There are twenty-one thousand six hundred breaths throughout a day and a night. This (repetition of *haṃsa* or *soham*) is called *Ajapā Gāyatrī*. The *jīva* always repeats it. -84.

मूलाऽऽधारे यथा हंसस्तथा हि हृदि पङ्कजे ।

तथा नासापुटद्वन्द्वे त्रिभिर्हंससमागमः ॥८५॥

mūlādhāre yathā haṃsastathā hi hṛdi paṅkaje /

tathā nāsāpuṭadvandve tribhirhaṃsasamāgamaḥ //85//

There are three places of in and out movements of the air (while repeating *haṃsa*). They are *mūlādhāra*, *anāhata*, and *nāsāpuṭa* (the two nostrils) which are the meeting points of *haṃsa*. -85.

षण्णवत्यङ्गुलीमानं शरीरं कर्मरूपकम् ।

देहाद्वहिर्गतो वायुः स्वभावात् द्वादशाङ्गुलिः ॥८६॥

गायने षोडशाङ्गुल्यो भोजने विंशतिस्तथा ।

चतुर्विंशाङ्गुलिः पन्थे निद्रायां त्रिंशदङ्गुलि ।

मैथुने षट्त्रिंशदुक्तं व्यायामे च ततोऽधिकम् ॥८७॥

ṣaṇṇavatyaṅgulīmānam śarīram karmarūpakam /

dehādvahirgato vāyuḥ svabhāvāt dvādśāṅguliḥ //86//

gāyane ṣoḍaśāṅgulyao bhojane vimśatistathā /

caturvimśāṅguli panthe nidrāyām triśadaṅguliḥ /

maithune ṣaṭtrimśaduktam vyāyāme ca tato'dhikam //87/

The physical body has the length of ninety-six *aṅgulas* (*aṅgula*, a measure of thumb's width) according to one's karma. The length of the out going air is normally twelve *aṅgulas*. During singing it is sixteen *aṅgulas* long. During eating it is twenty *aṅgulas* long. During walking it is twenty-four *aṅgulas* long. During sleep it is thirty *aṅgulas* long. During sexual intercourse it is thirty-six *aṅgulas* long and during physical exercise it is significantly longer than that. -86-

87.

स्वभावेऽस्य गतेर्न्यूने परमायुः प्रवर्धते ।

आयुःक्षयोऽधिके प्रोक्तो मारुतेचान्तराद्गते ॥८८॥

तस्मात्प्राणे स्थिते देहे मरणं नैव जायते ।

वायुना घटसम्बन्धे भवेत्केवलकुम्भकम् ॥८९॥

svabhāve'sya gaternyūne paramāyuḥ pravardhate /

āyuḥkṣayo'dhike prokto mārutecāntarādgate //88//

tasmātprāṇe sthite dehe maraṇam naiva jāyate /

vāyunā ghaṭasambandhe bhavet kevalakumbhakaḥ //89//

When the length of the out going breath is naturally decreased, longevity is increased. It is said that longevity decreases when there is a greater outward flow of *maruta* or *prāṇa*. Therefore, as long as *prāṇa* exists in the body, there is no death. When *prāṇa* is naturally restrained within the body, this is called *kevala kumbhaka*. -88-89.

यावज्जीवं जपेन्मन्त्रम् अजपासङ्ख्यकेवलम् ।

अद्यावधि धृतं सङ्ख्याविभ्रमं केवली कृते ॥९०॥

अत एव हि कर्तव्यः केवलीकुम्भको नरैः ।

केवली चाजपासङ्ख्या द्विगुणा च मनोन्मनी ॥९१॥

yāvajjīvam japenmantram ajapāsaṅkhyakevalam /

adhyāvadhi dhṛtam saṅkhyāvibhramam kevalī kṛte //90//

ata eva hi kartavyaḥ kevalīkumbhako naraiḥ /

kevalī cājapāsaṅkhyā dviguṇā ca manonmanī //91//

All *jīvas* are normally repeating certain numbers of *ajapā mantra* daily. As long as body exists, one should continue repeating *ajapā mantra* with counts while performing *kevalī kumbhaka*. When *kevalī* is done or twenty-one thousands six hundred repetitions are completed, the rate of respiration decreases and longevity increases. When the number of repetitions of *ajapā mantra* is doubled, there remains *kevalī* alone and a blissful state is achieved. Therefore, it is certainly a task of yogis to practice *kevalī kumbhaka*. -90-91.

नासाभ्यां वायुमाकृष्य केवलं कुम्भकं चरेत् ।

एकादिकचतुः षष्टिं धारयेत् प्रथमे दिने ॥९२॥

nāsābhyāṃ vāyumākṛṣya kevalaṃ kumbhakaṃ caret /

ekādikacatuḥ ṣaṣṭiṃ dhārayet prathame dine //92//

Inhaling air through both nostrils, naturally hold the breath by *kevalī kumbhaka*. Hold the breath (by this *kumbhaka*) from one to sixty-four times on the first day. -92.

केवलीमष्टधा कुर्याद्यामे यामे दिने दिने ।

अथवा पञ्चधा कुर्याद्यथा तत्कथयामि ते ॥९३॥

प्रातर्मध्याह्नसायाह्ने मध्ये रात्रिचतुर्थके ।

त्रिसन्ध्यमथवा कुर्यात्सममाने दिने दिने ॥९४॥

kevalīmaṣṭadhā kuryādyāme yāme dine dine /

athavā pañcadhā kuryādyathā tat kathayāmi te //93//

prātarmadhyāhnasāyāhne madhye rātricaturthake /

trisandhyamathavā kuryātsamamāne dine dine //94//

Kevalī kumbhaka should be practiced eight times, once every three hours a day or it should be practiced five times a day, as I explain: - in early morning, at noon, in twilight, at midnight and in the fourth quarter of the night. Or it should be practiced in *samamāna* (equal duration/length of time) three times a day at the *trisandhyās* (the three times of transitions or sunrise, noon and sunset). -93-94.

पञ्चवारं दिने वृद्धिर्वारैकं च दिने तथा ।

अजपापरिमाणं च यावत्सिद्धिः प्रजायते ॥९५॥

प्राणायामं केवलीं च तदा वदति योगवित् ।

केवलीकुम्भके सिद्धे किं न सिध्यति भूतले ॥९६॥

pañcavāraṃ dine vṛddhirvāraikaṃ ca dine tathā /

ajapāparimāṇaṃ ca yāvat siddhiḥ prājayate //95//

prāṇāyāmaṃ kevalīṃ ca tadā vadati yogavit /

kevalīkumbhake siddhe kiṃ na sidhyati bhūtale //96//

One should go on increasing the period/length of *ajapā japa* practice five times every day until the result of perfection is not achieved. One who knows *prāṇāyāma* and *kevalī* is called the knower of yoga. One who has gained mastery over *kevalī kumbhaka*, what cannot he achieve in this earth? -96.

इति श्रीघेरण्डसंहितायां घेरण्डचण्डसंवादे

प्राणायामप्रयोगो नाम पञ्चमोपदेशः ॥

iti śrīgheraṇḍasamhitāyāṃ gheraṇḍacaṇḍasamvāde

prāṇāyāmaprayogo nāma pañcamopadeśaḥ /

Thus ends the Fifth Chapter of *Gheraṇḍa Samhitā*

entitled *Prāṇāyāma* Practice.

Chapter Six

Discourse On Dhyāna

घेरण्ड उवाच ।

स्थूलं ज्योतिस्तथा सूक्ष्मं ध्यानस्य त्रिविधं विदुः ।

स्थूलं मूर्तिमयं प्रोक्तं ज्योतिस्तेजोमयं तथा ।

सूक्ष्मं बिन्दुमयं ब्रह्म कुण्डली परदेवता ॥१॥

gheraṇḍa uvāca /

sthūlaṃ jyotistathā sūkṣmam dhyānasya trividhaṃ viduḥ /

sthūlaṃ mūrtimayaṃ proktaṃ jyotistejomayaṃ tathā /

sūkṣmaṃ vindumayaṃ brahma kuṇḍalī paradevatā //1//

Sage *Gheraṇḍa* said: - *Sthūla* (gross), *jyoti* (light) and *sūkṣma* (subtle) are known three types of *dhyāna* (meditation). It is called *Sthūla dhyāna* (gross meditation) when one meditates on the physical form (of a guru, *devatā* or deity). It is *jyoti dhyāna* (meditation on light) when one meditates on the radiant form of *Brahma*, full of light. It is *sūkṣma dhyāna* (subtle meditation) when one meditates on *Brahma* in the form of *bindu* and *kuṇḍalī śakti*, the divine power. -1.

[105]

Sthūla Dhyāna

स्वकीयहृदये ध्यायेत्सुधासागरमुत्तमम् ।

तन्मध्ये रत्नद्वीपं तु सुरत्नवालुकामयम् ॥२॥

चतुर्दिक्षु नीपतरुं बहुपुष्पसमन्वितम् ।

नीपोपवनसङ्कुलैर्वेष्टितं परिखा इव ॥३॥

मालतीमल्लिकाजातीकेसरैश्चम्पकैस्तथा ।

पारिजातैः स्थलपद्मैर्गन्धामोदितदिङ्मुखैः ॥४॥

svakīyahṛdaye dhyāyet sudhāsāgaramuttamam /

tanmadhye ratnadvīpaṃ tu suratnavālukāmayam //2//

caturdikṣu nīpataruṃ bahupuṣpasamanvitam /

nipopavanasaṅkulairveṣṭitaṃ parikhā iva //3//

mālatīmallikājātikeśaraiścampakaistathā /

pārijātaiḥ sthalapadmairgandhāmoditadiṅmukhaiḥ //4//

Contemplate a magnificent ocean of nectar in the heart. In the middle of it, there is an island of precious jewels and the sand is made of the dust of diamonds and jewels. On all four sides *nīpataru* (a kind of tree, its flowers and fruits) trees are laden with many flowers. On the island these trees are surrounded like ditches by many varieties of flowering trees like *mālatī, mallikā, jāti, keśara, campaka, pārijāta* and *padma* (these are name of flowers), and their fragrance spreads every direction all over the island. -2-4.

तन्मध्ये संस्मरेद्योगी कल्पवृक्षं मनोहरम् ।

चतुःशाखाचतुर्वेदं नित्यपुष्पफलान्वितम् ॥५॥

भ्रमराः कोकिलास्तत्र गुञ्जन्ति निगदन्ति च ।

ध्यायेत्तत्र स्थिरो भूत्वा महामाणिक्यमण्डपम् ॥६॥

तन्मध्ये तु स्मरेद्योगी पर्यङ्कं सुमनोहरम् ।

तत्रेष्टदेवतां ध्यायेद्यद्ध्यानं गुरुभाषितम् ॥७॥

यस्य देवस्य यद्रूपं यथा भूषणवाहनम् ।

तद्रूपं ध्यायते नित्यं स्थूलध्यानमिदं विदुः ॥८॥

tanmadhyesamsmaredyogī kalpavṛkṣam manoharam /

catuhśākhācaturvedaṃ nityapuṣpaphalānvitam //5//

bhramarāḥ kokilāstatra guñjanti nigadanti ca /

dhyāyettatra sthiro bhūtvā mahāmāṇikyamaṇḍapam //6//

tanmadhye tu smaredyogī paryaṅkaṃ sumanoharam /

tatreṣṭadevatāṃ dhyāyet yatdhyānaṃ gurubhāṣitam //7//

yasya devasya yadrūpaṃ yathā bhūṣaṇavāhanam /

tadrūpaṃ dhyāyate nityaṃ sthuladhyānamidaṃ viduḥ //8//

A yogi should contemplate that in the middle of this island there is a beautiful *kalpa vṛkṣa* (wish fulfilling tree). The four branches of this tree represent the four *Vedas.* It is always laden with flowers and fruits. Wild bees make humming sounds and cuckoos sing with melodious voice there. There is a great pavilion made of precious gems and a throne decorated with jewels. On this throne contemplate the *deva* (deity) as per the teaching of the guru and always meditate on the form, jewelry and vehicle of the deity. This is called *sthula dhyāna.* -5-8.

Another Method

सहस्रारे महापद्मे कर्णिकायां विचिन्तयेत् ।

विलग्नसहितं पद्मं द्वादशैर्दलसंयुतम् ॥९॥

शुक्लवर्णं महातेजो द्वादशैर्बीजभाषितम् ।

हसक्षमलवरयुं हसखफ्रें यथाक्रमम् ॥१०॥

तन्मध्ये कर्णिकायां तु अकथादिरेखात्रयम् ।

हलक्षकोणसंयुक्तं प्रणवं तत्र वर्तते ॥११॥

sahasrāre mahāpadme karṇikāyaṃ vicintayet /

vilagnasahitaṃ padmaṃ dalairdvādaśabhiryutam //9//

śuklavarṇaṃ mahātejo dvādaśairbījabhāṣitam /

hasakṣamalavarayuṃ hasakhaprem yathākramam //10//

tanmadhye karṇikāyāṃ tu akathādi rekhātrayam /

halakṣakoṇasamyuktaṃ praṇavam tatra vartate //11//

Imagine that in the region of *sahasrāra* there is a great lotus with a thousand petals and in its center there is a small lotus with twelve petals. Its petals are white and full of radiance with the twelve shining *bīja mantras* located on them: *ha, sa, ksa, ma, la, va, ra, yum, ha, sa, kha* and *phrem*. In the center of this small lotus there are three lines *a, ka* and *tha* forming a triangle. This triangle has three angles with their symbols *ha, la* and *kṣa*. The *praṇava* (OM) is situated in the middle of this triangle. -9-11.

नादबिन्दुमयं पीठं ध्यायेत्तत्र मनोहरम् ।

तत्रोपरि हंसयुग्मं पादुका तत्र वर्तते ॥१२॥

nādavindumayaṃ pīṭhaṃ dhyāyettatra manoharam /

tatropari haṃsayugmaṃ pādukā tatra vartate //12//

Contemplate that in that thousand petalled lotus there is a beautiful seat with *nāda* (sound) and *bindu* (light). There are two swans (as symbol of *nāda* and *bindu*) and a pair of sandals on it (as symbol of the guru). -12.

ध्यायेत्तत्र गुरुं देवं द्विभुजं च त्रिलोचनम् ।

श्वेताम्बरधरं देवं शुक्लगन्धानुलेपनम् ॥१३॥

शुक्लपुष्पमयं माल्यं रक्तशक्तिसमन्वितम् ।

एवंविधगुरुध्यानात्स्थूलध्यानं प्रसिध्यति ॥१४॥

dhyāyettatra gurum devam dvibhujam ca trilocanam /

svetāmbaradharam devam śuklagandhānulepanam //13//

śuklapuṣpamayam mālyam raktaśaktisamanvitam /

evamvidhagurudhyānāt sthūladhyānam prasidhyati //14//

Now contemplate on the guru *deva*, having two arms and three eyes, wearing white clothes, a garland of whilte flowers and anointed with aromatic white sandalwood paste. On his left side there is his *śakti* in red color. By meditating on the guru in this way, perfection is attained in *sthūla dhyāna.* -13-14.

Jyoti Dhyāna

घेरण्ड उवाच ।

कथितं स्थूलध्यानं तु तेजोध्यानं श्रृणुष्व मे ।

यद्ध्यानेन योगसिद्धिरात्मप्रत्यक्षमेव च ॥१५॥

gheraṇda uvāca /

kathitam sthūla dhyānam tu tejodhyānam śruṇuṣva me /

yaddhyānena yogasiddhirātmapratyakṣameva ca //15//

Sage *Gheraṇda* said: - I have described you *sthūla dhyāna.* Now listen to *tejodhyāna* (the meditation on light). By this meditation one attains *yogasiddhi* (perfection in yoga) and gains a direct knowledge of the Self. -15.

मूलाधारे कुण्डलिनी भुजङ्गाकाररूपिणी ।

तत्र तिष्ठति जीवात्मा प्रदीपकलिकाकृतिः ।

[109]

ध्यायेत्तेजोमयं ब्रह्म तेजोध्यानं परात्परम् ॥१६॥

mūlādhāre kuṇḍalinī bhujaṅgākārarūpiṇīḥ /

tatra tiṣṭhati jīvātmā pradīpakalikākṛti /

dhyāyettejomayaṃ brahma tejodhyānaṃ parātparam //16//

Kuṇḍalinī rests in *mūlādhāra* in the form of a serpent. *Jīvātmā* (the embodied Self) remains there like the flame of a lamp. Meditate on the luminous *Brahma* there. This is the supreme *tejodhyāna* or *jyoti dhyāna* (meditation on light).-16.

भ्रुवोर्मध्ये मनोर्ध्वे च यत्तेज: प्रणवात्मकम् ।

ध्यायेत् ज्वालावलीयुक्तं तेजोध्यानं तदेव हि ॥१७॥

bhruvormadhye manordve yattejaḥ praṇavātmakam /

dhyāyet jvālāvalīyuktaṃ tejodhyānaṃ tadeva hi //17//

Between the eyebrows, above the area of *manas* (the mind) there is light in the form of *praṇava* (OM). Meditate on this flaming light. This is verily called *tejodhyāna*. -17.

Sūkṣma Dhyāna

घेरण्ड उवाच ।

तेजोध्यानं श्रृतं चण्ड सूक्ष्मध्यानं श्रृणुष्व मे ।

बहुभाग्यवशाद्यस्य कुण्डली जाग्रती भवेत् ॥१८॥

आत्मना सह योगेन नेत्ररन्ध्राद्विनिर्गता ।

विहरेद्राजमार्गे च चञ्चलत्वान्न दृश्यते ॥१९॥

gheraṇḍa uvāca /

tejodhyānaṃ śrutaṃ caṇḍa sūkṣmadhyānaṃ śruṇuṣva me /

bahubhāgyavaśādyasya kuṇḍalī jāgrati bhavet //18//

[110]

ātmanā saha yogena netrarandhrādvinirgatā /

viharedrājamārge ca cañcalatvānna dṛśyate //19//

Sage *Gheraṇḍa* said: - O *Caṇḍa*, you have heard the *tejodhyāna*, now listen to *sūkṣma dhyāna* (subtle meditation). One whose *kuṇḍalinī śhakti* is awakened by the power of great fortune, it unites with *Ātmā* and goes upward through *netra randhra* (the holes/openings of the eyes) and roams on the *rajamārga* (high way). It is not visible because of its (subtle) restlessness. -18-19.

शाम्भवीमुद्रया योगी ध्यानयोगेन सिध्यति ।

सूक्ष्मध्यानमिदं गोप्यं देवानामपि दुर्लभम् ॥२०॥

sāmbhavīmudrayā yogī dhyānayogena sidhyati /

sūkṣmadhyānamidaṃ gopyaṃ devānāpi durlabham //20//

A yogi attains *siddhi* (perfection) through the practice of *sāmbhavī mudrā* and *dhyāna yoga* (meditation on *kuṇḍalinī śhakti*). This is called *sūkṣma dhyāna* which is secret. It is difficult to obtain even by gods. -20.

स्थूलध्यानाच्छतगुणं तेजोध्यानं प्रचक्षते ।

तेजोध्यानाल्लक्षगुणं सूक्ष्मध्यानं परात्परम् ॥२१॥

sthūladhyānācchataguṇaṃ tejodhyānaṃ pracakṣate /

tejodhyānāllakṣaguṇaṃ sūkṣmadhyānaṃ parātparam //21//

Tejodhyāna (meditation on light) is a hundred times superior to *sthūla dhyāna* (meditation on form) and *sūkṣma dhya*na (subtle meditation) is a hundred thousand times superior to *tejodhyānā.* -21.

इति ते कथितं चण्ड ध्यानयोगं सुदुर्लभम् ।

आत्मा साक्षात् भवेद्यस्मात्तस्माद्ध्यानं विशिष्यते ॥२३॥

iti te kathitaṃ caṇḍa dhyānayogaṃ sudurlabham /

ātmasākṣād bhaved yasmāttasmāddhyānaṃ viśiṣyate //22//

O *Caṇḍa*! Thus, I have told you the *dhyānayoga* which is extremely difficult to obtain. Knowledge of the Self becomes direct by its practice. Therefore, this *dhyānayoga* is uniquely admired. -22.

इति श्रीघेरण्डसंहितायां घेरण्डचण्डसंवादे

ध्यानयोगो नाम षष्ठोपदेशः ॥

iti śrīgheraṇḍasamhitāyāṃ gheraṇḍacaṇḍasamvāde

dhyānayogo nāma ṣaṣṭhopadeśaḥ /

Thus ends the Sixth Chapter of *Gheraṇḍa Samhitā*

entitled Dhyānayoga.

Chapter Seven

Discourse On Samādhi

घेरण्ड उवाच ।

समाधिश्च परो योगो बहुभाग्येन लभ्यते ।

गुरोः कृपाप्रसादेन प्राप्यते गुरुभक्तितः ॥१ ॥

gheraṇḍa uvāca /

samādhiśca paro yogo bahubhāgyena labhyate /

guroḥ kṛpāprasādena prāpyate gurubhaktitaḥ //1//

Sage *Gheraṇḍa* said: - *Samādhi* is the supreme yoga and is attained by great fortunate. It is received through the compassion and grace of the gurus by earnest devotion to them. -1.

विद्याप्रतीतिः स्वगुरुप्रतीतिः

आत्मप्रतीतिर्मनसः प्रबोधः ।

दिने दिने यस्य भवेत्स योगी

सुशोभनाभ्यासमुपैति सद्यः ॥२ ॥

vidyāpratītiḥ svagurupratītiḥ

ātmapratītirmanasaḥ prabodhaḥ /

dine dine yasya bhavetsa yogī

suśobhanābhyāsamupaiti sadyaḥ //2//

The yogi is quickly endowed with this auspicious practice of *Samādhi* who has the insight of knowledge, has faith in his guru, has faith in his Self and has an awakening mind everyday. -2.

घटाद्भिन्नं मनः कृत्वा ऐक्यं कुर्यात्परात्मनि ।

समाधिं तं विजानीयात् मुक्तसंज्ञो दशादिभिः ॥३॥

ghaṭādbhinnaṃ manaḥ kṛtvā

aikyaṃ kuryātparamātmani /

samādhiṃ taṃ vijānīyān

muktasaṅjñyo daśādibhi //3//

A yogi should separate his mind from the body and unite it with *paramātmā* (the Supreme Soul). This should be known as *Samādhi*, a free state of consciousness from all conditions. -3.

अहं ब्रह्म न चान्योऽस्मि ब्रह्मैवाहं न शोकभाक् ।

सच्चिदानन्दरूपोऽहं नित्यमुक्तः स्वभाववान् ॥४॥

ahaṃ brahma na cānyo'smi

brahmaivāhaṃ na śokabhāk /

saccidānandarūpo'haṃ

nityamuktaḥ svabhāvavān //4//

I am *Brahma*. I am not anything else. I am *Brahma* alone. I am not the possessor of sorrow. I am the form of *Sat, Cit* and *Ānanda* (*Saccidānanda* – Truth-Consciousness-Bliss). I am ever free and exist in my own nature. -4.

शाम्भव्या चैव भ्रामर्या खेचर्या योनिमुद्रया ।

ध्यानं नादं रसानन्दं लयसिद्धिश्चतुर्विधा ॥५॥

पञ्चधा भक्तियोगेन मनोमूर्च्छा च षड्विधा ।

षड्विधोऽयं राजयोगः प्रत्येकमवधारयेत् ॥६॥

śambhavyā caiva bhrāmaryā khecaryā yonimudrayā /

dhyānaṃ nādaṃ rasānandaṃ layasiddhiścaturvidhā //5//

pañcadhā bhaktiyogena manomūrcchā ca ṣaḍvidhā /

ṣaḍvidho 'yaṃ rājayogaḥ pratyekamavadhārayet //6//

The four types of *samādhi: dhyāna, nāda, rasānanda* and *laya* are accomplished by *śambhavī, khecari, bhrāmari* and *yoni mudrās. Bhaktiyoga* (yoga of devotion) *samādhi* is the fifth and *manomūrcchā samādhi* is the sixth. These are the six types of *samādhis* in *Rajayoga.* On should practice each of them in order. -5-6.

Dhyānayoga Samādhi

शाम्भवीं मुद्रिका: कृत्वा आत्मप्रत्यक्षमानयेत् ।

बिन्दु ब्रह्ममयं दृष्ट्वा मनस्तत्र नियोजयेत् ॥७॥

śāmbhavīṃ mudrikāḥ kṛtvā ātmapratyakṣamānayet /

bindubrahmamayaṃ dṛṣṭvā manastatra niyojayet //7//

Assuming *śāmbhavī mudrā,* perceive the Self. Having seen the *bindu* in the form of *Brahma,* concentrate the mind there. -7.

खमध्ये कुरु चात्मानमात्ममध्ये च खं कुरु ।

आत्मानं खमयं दृष्ट्वा न किञ्चिदपि बुध्यते ।

सदानन्दमयो भूत्वा समाधिस्थो भवेन्नरः ॥८॥

khamadhye kurucātmānamātmamadhye ca khaṃ kuru /

ātmānaṃ khamayaṃ dṛtvā na kiñcidapi budhyate /

sadānandamayo bhūtvā samādhistho bhavennaraḥ //8//

Dissolve the Self in the eternal space and the space in the Self. Perceiving the *Ātmā* full of space or *Brahma,* nothing else is seen (except *Brahma*). Being ever full of bliss, a person is established in *samādhi.* -8.

Nādayoga Samādhi

अनिलं मन्दवेगेन भ्रामरीकुम्भकं चरेत् ।

मन्दं मन्दं रेचयेद्वायुं भृङ्गनादं ततो भवेत् ॥९॥

अन्तःस्थं भ्रमरीनादं श्रृत्वा तत्र मनो नयेत् ।

समाधिर्जायते तत्र आनन्दः सोऽहमित्यतः ॥१०॥

anilaṃ mandavegena bhrāmarīkumbhakaṃ caret /

mandaṃ mandaṃ recayedvāyuṃ bhṛṅganādaṃ tato bhavet //9//

antaḥsthaṃ bhramarīnādaṃ śrutvā tatra mano nayet /

samādhirjāyate tatra cānandaḥ so'hamityataḥ //10//

Inhaling the air in a slow speed, perform *bhrāmarī kumbhaka.* Exhale the air slowly and slowly. This slow exhalation creates a sound of a wild bee. Listening to this internal sound of *bhramara* (the wild bee), focus the mind there. By this, a *samādhi* with a blissful state occurs there with the knowledge of 'I am That'. -9-10.

Rasanānanda Samādhi

खेचरीमुद्रासाधनात् रसनोर्ध्वगता यदा ।

तदा समाधिसिद्धिः स्याद्धित्वा साधारणक्रियाम् ॥११॥

khecarimudrāsādhanāt rasanordvagatā yadā /

tadā samādhisiddhiḥ syāddhitvā sadhāraṇakriyām //11//

When the tongue is turned upward through the perfection of *khecari mudrā*, then by this simple yogic practice one attains *siddhi* in *samādhi*. -11.

Layasiddhi Samādhi

योनिमुद्रां समासाद्य स्वयं शक्तिमयो भवेत् ।

सुश्रृङ्गाररसेनैव विहरेत्परमात्मनि ॥१२॥

आनन्दमयः सम्भूत्वा ऐक्यं ब्रह्मणि सम्भवेत् ।

अहं ब्रह्मेति चाद्वैतसमाधिस्तेन जायते ॥१३॥

yonimudrāṃ samāsadya svayaṃ śaktimayo bhavet /
suśṛṅgārarasenaiva viharetparamātmani //12//
ānandamayaḥ sambhūtvā ekyaṃ brahmaṇi sambhavet /
ahaṃ brahmeti cādvaitasamādhistena jāyate //13//

After properly perfecting *yoni mudrā*, a yogi should imagine that he himself is full of *Śakti* and *Paramātmā*. Then again feel that in him and in *Paramātmā* (the Supreme Soul) *Śakti* and *Puruṣa* are roaming joyfully. After being established in a blissful oneness, he becomes united with *Brahma* and declares that 'I am *Brahma*'. This is called *advaita* (non-dual) *samādhi* or *laya siddhi samādhi*. -12-13

Bhaktiyoga Samādhi

स्वकीयहृदये ध्यायेदिष्टदेव स्वरूपकम् ।

चिन्तयेद्भक्तियोगेन परमाह्लादपूर्वकम् ॥१४॥

आनन्दाश्रुपुलकेन दशाभावः प्रजायते ।

समाधिः सम्भवेत्तेन सम्भवेच्च मनोन्मनी ॥१५॥

svakīyahṛdaye dhyāyediṣṭadeva svarūpakam /
cintayedbhaktiyogena paramāhlādapūrvakam //14//

ānandāśrupulakena daśābhāvaḥ prajāyate /

samādhiḥ sambhavettena sambhavecca manonmanī //15//

Imagine the form of *iṣṭadeva* (the favorable god) in the heart and meditate on it with supreme joy and highest devotion. This brings a state of bliss with tears and a sign of rapture (with erection of hairs) in the body. This gives rise to *samādhi* and *manonmanī* (a state similar to *samādhi*). -14-15.

Manomūrcchā Samādhi

मनोमूर्च्छां रागाराध्य मन आत्मनि योजयेत् ।

परात्मनः समायोगात्समाधिं समवाप्नुयात् ॥१६॥

manomūrcchāṃ samāsādya mana ātmani yojayet /

paramātmanaḥ samāyogātsamādhiṃ samavāpnuyāt //16//

After perfecting *manomūrcchā kumbhaka*, one should meditate on *Ātmā*. By means of this, union with the *Paramātma* is attained in *samādhi*. -16.

Greatness of Samādhi Yoga

इति ते कथितं चण्ड समाधिर्मुक्तिलक्षणम् ।

राजयोगः समाधिः स्यादेकात्मन्येव साधनम् ।

उन्मनी सहजावस्था सर्वे चैकात्मवाचकाः ॥१७॥

iti te kathitaṃ caṇḍa samādhirmuktilakṣaṇam /

rājayogasamādhiḥ syādekātmanyeva sādhanam /

unmanī sahajāvasthā sarvecaikātmavācakā //17//

O *Caṇḍa*! I have explained you *samādhi* as a sign of *mukti* (liberation). This *Rājayoga samādhi* is one of the means of self-realization. *Unmanī* and *sahaja avasthā* are the same states of *samādhi* like *Rājayoga samādhi* with regard to the achievement of union with

[118]

Ātmā (the Self). So, they are all synonymous. -17.

जले विष्णुः स्थले विष्णुर्विष्णुः पर्वतमस्तके ।

ज्वालामालाकुले विष्णुः सर्वं विष्णुमयं जगत् ॥१८॥

jale viṣṇuḥ sthale viṣṇurviṣṇuḥ parvatamastake /

jvālāmālākule viṣṇuḥ sarva viṣṇumayaṃ jagat //18//

Lord *Viṣṇu* is in the water, Lord *Viṣṇu* is on land, Lord *Viṣṇu* is on the top of mountain, and Lord *Viṣṇu* is in the flames of fire. So, this whole universe is composed of Lord *Viṣṇu*. -18.

भूचराः खेचराश्चामी यावन्तो जीवजन्तवः ।

वृक्षगुल्मलतावल्लीतृणाद्या वारिपर्वताः ।

सर्वं ब्रह्म विजानीयात्सर्वं पश्यति चात्मनि ॥१९॥

bhūcarāḥ khecarāścāmī yāvanto jīvajantavaḥ /

vṛkṣagulmalatāvallītṛṣṇādyāḥ vāri parvatāḥ /

sarvaṃ brahma vijānīyātsarvaṃ paśyati cātmani //19//

All living creatures on earth, in air, trees, bushes, creepers, grass, oceans, mountains should be known as *Brahma*. One should see all in *Ātmā* (the Self) and *Ātmā* (the Self) in all. -19.

आत्मा घटस्थचैतन्यमद्वैतं शाश्वतं परम् ।

घटाद्विभिन्नतो ज्ञात्वा वीतरागं विवासनम् ॥२०॥

ātmā ghaṭasthacaitanyamadvaitaṃ śāśvataṃ param /

gaṭādvibhinnato jñātvā vītarāgaṃ vivāsanam //20//

One should consider that *Caitanya* (the Conscious Self) based in the body is non-dual (without a second), eternal and supreme. Knowing that *Ātmā* (the Self) or *Caitanya* (the Conscious Self) is separate from the body, one should be detached from worldly attachments and passions. -20.

एवं मिथः समाधिः स्यात्सर्वसङ्कल्पवर्जितः ।

स्वदेहे पुत्रदारादिबान्धवेषु धनादिषु ।

सर्वेषु निर्ममो भूत्वा समाधिं समवाप्नुयात् ॥२१॥

evaṃ mithaḥ samādhiḥ syātsarvasaṅkalpavarjitaḥ /

svadehe putradārādibāndhaveṣu dhanādiṣu /

sarveṣu nirmamo bhūtvā samādhi samavāpnuyāt //21//

Thus, *samādhi* should be attained departing from all desires and attachments of the body, son, spouse, relatives, wealth and treasure, etc. Keeping the mind free from all worldly desires, try to achieve *samādhi*. -21.

तत्त्वं लयामृतं गोप्यं शिवोक्तं विविधानि च ।

तेषां सङ्क्षेपमादाय कथितं मुक्तिलक्षणम् ॥२२॥

tattvaṃ layāmṛtaṃ gopyaṃ śivoktaṃ vividhāni ca /

teṣāṃ saṅkṣepamādāya kathitam muktilakṣaṇam /22//

A variety of this secret *Laya Amṛta Tattva* (essence of absorption in nectar) has been expounded by Lord *Śiva*. I have explained you briefly with regard to it as a sign of liberation. -22.

इति ते कथितं चण्ड समाधि दुर्लभः परः ।

यं ज्ञात्वा न पुनर्जन्म जायते भूमि मण्डले ॥२३॥

iti te kathitaṃ caṇḍa samādhi durlabhaḥ paraḥ /

yaṃ jñātvā na punarjanma jāyate bhūmi maṇḍale //23//

O *Caṇḍa*! Thus I have told you about *samādhi* which is supreme and difficult to attain. By knowing this, one is not born again in this terrestrial world. -23.

इति श्रीघेरण्डसंहितायां घेरण्डचण्डसंवादे

[120]

समाधियोगो नाम सप्तमोपदेशः ॥

iti śrīgheraṇḍasamhitāyāṃ gheraṇḍacaṇḍasaṃvāde
samādhiyogo nāma saptamopadeśaḥ /
Thus ends the Seventh Chapter of *Gheraṇḍa Samhitā*
entitled *Samādhi Yoga.*

A Key to Transliteration

<u>Vowels</u>

अ आ इ ई उ ऊ ऋ ॠ

a ā i ī u ū ṛ ṝ

लृ ॡ ए ऐ ओ औ अं अः

lṛ lṝ e ai o au aṃ aḥ

<u>Consonants</u>

क ख ग घ ङ - Gutturals:

ka kha ga gha ṅa

च छ ज झ ञ - Palatals:

ca cha ja jha ña

ट ठ ड ढ ण - Cerebrals:

ṭa ṭha ḍa ḍha ṇa

त थ द ध न - Dentals:

ta tha da dha na

प फ ब भ म - Labials:

pa pha ba bha ma

य र ल व - Semivowels:

ya ra la va

श ष स ह   - Sibilants:

śa ṣa sa ha

क्ष त्र ज्ञ   - Compound Letters:

kṣa tra jña

Aspirate: ह - ha, Anusvara: अं - aṃ,

Visharga - aḥ - अः

Unpronounced अ - a - ऽ - ', आ - ā - ऽऽ - ''

Also by This Author

Yoga Kundalini Upanishad (in English)

Yoga Darshana Upanishad (in English)

Minor Yoga Upanishads (in English)

Dattatreya Yogashastra (in English)

Hatha Yoga Pradipika (in English)

Yogatattva Upanishad (in English)

Triyoga Upanishad (in English)

Dviyoga Samhita (in English)

Shiva Samhita (in English)

Shiva Samhita (in Nepali)

Surya Namskara (in Nepali)

Durga Strotram (in Nepali)

Vagalamukhi Stotram (in Nepali)

Amogha Śivakavacham (in Nepali)